THE GIFT OF DEPRESSION

My Little Scrap Book

BOB EDEN

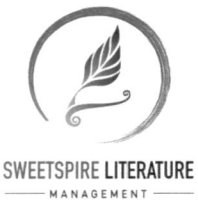

SWEETSPIRE LITERATURE
—— MANAGEMENT ——

Contents

Introduction

G'day folks and welcome to "The Gift of Depression, My Little Scrap Book". Not sure about what is a normal gestation period for a book, but this has taken many years to come out!

As all are S U E, Sovereign Unique and Equal, I knew I could not write a How-to book so what follows is just my story, my journey from trauma and despair to contentment and some insights and tools I picked up along the way.

My life is simple now for I live in Heartspace , hence the format of the book is simple , innocent and sometimes chaotic but that is just how my journey unfolded, K I S S: Keep It Simple Sovereign.

My intention is ,that anyone reading this little missive will come away feeling lifted in some way and with the hope that there is a pathway through depression that is natural and drug free.

I AM just a simple bloke, and if I can do it, so can others. Once I realised that my depression was a wound of the soul and had nothing to do with my mind, the pathway became clear,

So here it is warts and all!

Injoy, Bob and Charlie (That's my dog).

Foreword

By David Richards:
https://www.davidrichardsauthor.com/

Bob Eden was the first person ever to reach out to me after I launched my website in support of the launch of my second book, The Lighthouse Keeper. It was January of 2020 when he sent me an email.

He shared his story and, while we grew up in completely different worlds, his story was easy enough to relate to. I'll share a bit of my own in reflection:

Growing up on military bases for most of my life, I have come to appreciate the sharp contrast between living on a military base and living in the civilian world. I went to a high school on base, surrounded by other military dependants (the military's term for people not wearing the uniform but nonetheless dependent on those who do), people on base didn't lock their doors. Military police vehicles were a common site in our neighbourhoods. They were Marines protecting Marines and their families. Serious crime was virtually nonexistent.

Marines were everywhere. In the cars that you drove past. At the grocery store. At the beach!

After living out of uniform for fifteen years, well, I see that life as a civilian is different. Not only is it different; I am in quite the minority, as the latest estimates put the total number of people currently serving in the military worldwide at somewhere less than 30 million people. 30 million out of a planet of seven and a half billion people. By comparison, 300 million people saw combat during World War Two, with several other million serving in countries that were not directly engaged in the combat (the world population in 1940 was 2.3 billion).

My relationship with the military is a bit of a tangled mess. Growing up, I deeply resented the Marines, and my father especially, for all the moves and friendships that ended before I wanted them to. It makes perfect sense then, that I would choose the military as a career. If I am going to make myself miserable, I might as well get paid to do it! seemed to be my thinking at the time. The truth was, I wanted to write yet lacked the confidence and wisdom to understand what it meant to pursue one's dreams.

At the same time, the military is literally a part of my DNA; I would not be who I am today had I not gone through everything I did, in and out of uniform. The military has a knack for tearing people down, only to transform them into something greater. More than anything though, the military lights a peculiar spark inside people; it may come in the form of a drill instructor roaring from his diaphragm with enough vibrato to rattle windows, or when a leader you respect makes eye contact with you right before you're about to embark on a dangerous mission. It is the undeniable truth that there is someone inside you worth fighting for. That you have something to give to the world, and that if you work hard enough and dig deep enough, you're going to find that person.

We all want to be a better version of the person we currently are. If you aren't a little uncomfortable everyday, you aren't growing. That may be the biggest lesson I have taken away from the pandemic. It's easy to come up with excuses, or kick that can down the road. There's always tomorrow, right?

It takes courage to turn inward and figure out which beliefs are holding you back.

When Bob reached out to me recently ,to share he had put his book together and ask if I would write the foreword, I was honoured and elated. Honoured that anything I had written in either of my two books had meant something to another human being on this planet. Elated in that he had turned the lessons from his life into a triumph to be shared with others. I'm certain he hopes his story will touch at least one person's life.

Bob, mission accomplished!

David Richards
Cary, NC, USA

My Story

'The Wounds and Lessons of Childhood"

I was born in 1952, in England, very premature and delivered by cesarean section. My mother never forgave me for the scar on her belly. I was about 2lbs at birth and was not expected to live, but I did I AM a survivor!

Not sure why I chose my family. Mum was prone to violent outbursts of rage so if I got in range then I got hit whether I had been good or bad, so basically I got the crap beaten out of me for many years. So the message I internalised at that time was "Mum is often beating me, therefore she does not love me, I must be unlovable and it is all my fault!" and also "The World is not a Safe Place!"

Dad was a mythical being who was always at work, he came home after I went to bed and left for work before I came down for breakfast, so the message I got from Dad was " Dad never spends any time with me, therefore he does not love me, so I must be unlovable, and it is all my fault".

When I was six, Dad disappeared completely, he had a nervous breakdown and committed himself to Fairmile Hospital in Wallingford. I went to see him when I was nine and by that time he was institutionalised, just wandering around muttering phrases that he heard. He did not need electric shock therapy, he just needed a holiday!

To take the spotlight off my crazy family, Mum a Rage -aholic and Dad a Workaholic, I became the people pleaser and totally abandoned my needs to please others, a habit that I took into adulthood!

When I was about three it felt like someone had given me a wheelbarrow and so I started pushing it. I was young and strong so it was Ok! But as I moved through life, more junk was dumped into it, like my childhood abuse, socio-cultural conditioning , the indoctrination of the education system and all the rest of our societies constraints, until such time as it got to heavy to push anymore. That time was 1984, when at 3 am I had my first panic attack and began my dance with depression.

I couldn't understand it, I could not think my way out of it. I had a great job with Esso in research, was living the ideal magazine life, wife two kids, detached house, holidays in France, So what happened? And so the cycle of medications and psychologists and psychiatrists began and continued for many years.

Skipping back to childhood to keep things chronological. "When did I first start disbelieving in me?" My earliest recollection: I was about five years old and woke up one Sunday morning, got dressed and put on my favourite tee shirt, The Red One! So I went down for breakfast and Mum looked at me and said , Go and change, put on your blue tee shirt, you know that is your favourite! I got up , puzzled and went upstairs and changed, very confused, but MUM must be right and she is very big and I must not make her angry. That began a process of similar events and slowly I chopped more bits off me to fit into society, a habit I carried well into my forties!

So, how did I dig myself out of this hole?

My family and I emigrated to Australia in November 1989, for a fresh start? But after 13 years of working so hard, we realised we had become strangers and that our marriage was as shallow as the rest of my life. After a lot of soul searching we agreed to part and Pam and the kids went back to the UK. I stayed, I knew at some level this is where I AM meant to be. I must have cried for 6 months but had great support from friends I met in the Folk scene in Perth. Got a good job in automotive research and started rebuilding, but still with the old survival behaviours in place! My intellect was having a ball working in research, I was developing a following in the Folk Scene and playing in many bands in Perth and began touring in WA when work permitted, but my heart was heavy and I was still fighting with depression, it would be many years before I turned that fight into a dance!

Living in Freo, I got involved in personal growth and eventually became a counsellor. The first course I took was an ACA twelve step course for Adult children of Absent Parents which was very helpful up to a point where you have to surrender to god, I knew then that this was a parting of the ways. Next I did a course on anger management because Mum had all the anger, so I never learnt how to deal with it. About 1993 I came across John Bradshaw's work on the Inner Child and Family of Origin and was so Impressed that with my partner we bought all the tapes and used to run weekly group sessions. John's work opened the flood gates for me as I began to understand what my dysfunctional childhood had produced. I suppose it was at this time started to develop my sense of "Noticing" or "Awareness". Depression was still rolling in and out and one day I realised that medication only lasts for a couple of months and then produces the same symptoms it is supposed to cure and with my continued research into depression and mental illness I realised that not one psychologist or psychiatrist has ever cured any one, all they can do is work with the mind, medicate the pain and provide coping skills to handle the pain.

I think it was Jesse Greene in Freo who gave me this phrase: "If you don't hand it back, you pass it on!" I let that bubble for a while and then one day I sat down and wrote THE letter to Mum!

Dear Mum, I am writing to you to tell you how it felt for me growing up in our family. This is not about blame, just telling you my story, look forward to hearing yours, your loving son Bob.

And so I sat down and wrote and wrote about how I hated being hit so often or how she never came to school sports days, how she kept reminding me of the scar on her belly, any way. what I thought would be one or two pages turned into another WAR and PEACE but at least I got it all out. I posted this epic to Mum back in the UK and that was the hardest thing I had ever done, but I knew it was the way forward for I was being torn apart by " I hate my Mum for what She did to me, but you have to love your MUM!" this quandary was tearing my soul apart!

Six months later I get a reply, I am so sorry Bobby, you must think I am the worst mother in the world. I replied, no Mum I am just sharing my story, tell me yours! Time passes, a lot of it, then finally a letter from Mum arrives and she shares her story. She was born in 1924 in Germany between the wars her Dad was an alcoholic and her mum was a control freak, her cousins joined the SS or they were shot, it was a pretty horrific childhood and the I realised that Mum was just passing on what had been dumped on her and with that understanding I was able to move from hate back to a place of love,

and I felt so much lighter for that. A couple of days later, once I had stopped crying, I phoned Mum in England to learn that she was back in hospital with a second bout of bowel cancer, so I contacted the hospital and managed to speak to MUM and that was the first time and the last time we spoke as Mother and Son as adult to adult, so with tears at both sides of the pond we talked ! Two days later Mum passed away and I was so glad we had come to a loving closure.

A few days went by and I AM feeling much lighter but there is still a little niggle in my shoulders, still a heaviness there, then BOOM! Dad ya Bastard! So I got out the note pad and wrote a letter to DAD. Dad had died awhile back, not sure where or when, so I put the letter in an envelope and addressed it to DAD in Heaven and burnt it! Feeling much lighter now!

It was 1995 or 6, my mind was having a ball but my soul was crying, depression was still ruling the roost. I was performing at Araluen

Festival and there was a kombi for sale, so I bought it for 3 grand, got it back home fitted a pop top and set it up for the mobile life and I was ready! I remember going to my boss and saying " Chris I fear that if I lose this job I will die, so I quit" He was aware of my state of dis- ease, his reply was great, yeah Bob I kinda get that!

I put my house on the market and anything that would not suit the Kombi life, I sold or gave away, the first item being the TV! YAY!. Whilst waiting for the house to sell I planned my tour of the Folk Festivals and once the money was in the bank I was off. Don't get me wrong, I only realised about 35 grand from the sale of the house but it did fund my first tour. So I set of across Australia 40 days and 40 Nights springs to mind, it was the first time in my life that I had to spend time with me. It was a true right of passage. I would arrive at each festival a week or so early and join the volunteers who set up the festival and in the evenings I would sit with others around the campfire and share the music that I love. In this way, the people running the festival got to know what I was about musically! Next year, when I applied to perform at these festivals I got accepted as a paid performer, and so the wheel went round, about 8 times over 10 years . At the end of each tour I would generally return to Freo and Volunteer on the Leeuwin 2 a sail training vessel and sail up and down the west coast of Australia. Eventually "MOO" the kombi Died and I found myself in QLD. Got a job working on the boats in the Whitsundays and eventually became a commercial skipper and then a briefer. I AM now retired, living on my boat with my family, Barnaby and Charlie and I AM Content. I have created my dream for I AM Master and Commander of My Life.

I spent the first 40 years of my life chopping off bits of me to fit in and the remainder going back and gathering them all up for I now know that all of me is OK. I realised that I AM the only expert on my life and that the pain of depression was the pain of humanity having to live in such a crazy society and so I started the dance which is now over. My basic steps have been:

1. Empty the wheelbarrow
2. Question everything that does not resonate with my heart.
3. Deprogram myself from all the conditioning especially codependent behaviour
4. Re-establish my belief in me
5. Follow my Heart
6. Trust my In-Tuition!
7. Giggle a lot!

Simple really, any questions?

My Writings

"Simply Thank you"

After more than twenty years of fighting depression, many psychologists and many psychiatrists and so many cycles of medication, this simple personal insight brought me home!

To all those beautiful people who have suffered from depression I would like to say"Thank you, Simply Thank you" for doing such a wonderful job. Thank you for being such beautiful and courageous messengers, such shining beacons!

I hear your pain, I have felt your pain, and now I hear your message and I hear it loud and clear for your message is simply the pain of humanity and the way it has to live now. The way we are living now is so wrong, so wrong, there is so little human-ness left in the way we live. We need to change, and we need to change now! So now relax in the knowing of a job well done, your message has been heard, that there has never been anything wrong with you, you are simply a gifted messenger!

I know that place you go to; that deepening, darkening tunnel, which you shuffle down with trembling knees, and your body full of terror and panic. I know that place you go to, where the tunnel ends, where your bare feet are on solid ground but your toes are dangling over nothingness, an empty abyss, and it is so dark and frightening. Then dimly just ahead there is a feint outline, misty at first, that slowly forms into a shape, a doorway, and it's only about five feet away.

And I know that moment when you are rocking on the balls of your feet, trying to decide whether to jump or not."I wonder if I can leap across in one bound or shall I take a few steps back and take a running jump?"

Then for some reason, you stop rocking and plant your heels firmly back on the ground, and from somewhere deep, deep inside you grab hold of something primal, something essential and you turn around facing back the way you came and take a deep breath. I thank you in this moment for choosing to return to life rather than taking the leap of death.

All ahead is blackness and you squint your eyes and then dimly perceive a minute spec of light, so small you are not sure it is real at all. So you slowly retrace your steps, and that little spec of light gets bigger and bigger as you shuffle fearfully upwards.

You are heading back to the light and it is your light, and it is getting brighter and brighter until it's the colour of Cornish Ice cream and you can feel it's warmth enfold you, and suddenly you are out of the tunnel, back in the gallery of life.

So you take your light and sit down, and relax and look back at where you came from. The tunnel is gone, the entrance has been bricked over, then plastered over and some artists have painted a mural over the place honouring the purpose of the tunnel.

You are Home, you are safe! Well done and Simply Thank you! Namaste' Bob and Barnaby Eden. Woof.

"Rite of Passage".

It was about 8 years ago, about 7:30 at night.

I was on my boat Fidelio with Barnaby in Pioneer Bay. It was a lovely still evening and a full moon was rising, and the earth was still.

8

I was sitting on my bunk, typing on Facebook (Barnaby's Facebook page) when all of a sudden the lights went dim and I could not breathe. I looked across at the voltmeter 12.8 volts, so no problems there. Then I noticed, just at the edge of my vision, on the left hand side, a black, wispy ethereal presence. I said to myself"Hello old friend" for I had seen it before, I thought it was the grim reaper come to get me and that it was all over red rover!

I Still couldn't breathe, there was no pain and time seemed to be standing still. So I typed into facebook"If I do not post anything else in the next 30 minutes could someone please call marine rescue and come and get Barnaby" I did not panic, but just checked in with me, then I stood up, went up on deck and naked I jumped into the sea.

Pioneer bay is surrounded by mangrove trees, where crocodiles live, it was dark and that is when sharks and croc's feed. I lay on my back and spread out like a big starfish and was looking up at the sky. I could see two full moons, and then, all of a sudden, a huge gasp and I was breathing again! and that was the night I consciously bet my life on trusting my Intuition, my Inner Knowing. It was that night that I finally knew I had regained my faith in me. If you have not faced your own death, how can you really appreciate life, hey?

"Being / Doing"

Over the last 20 years or so I have slowly come to the realisation that I AM a human BEING and not a human DOING! and that just by simply BEING I AM DOING all the DOING i need to just to simply BE! My BEING consists of Being Authentic! Being Honourable! Being Honest! Simple Really!

"Re-Evaluation".

I hear a lot of folks saying"We need a revolution", Well I don't agree, when the changes comes, it will be gentle, It will not be a revolution but simply a Re-Evaluation by the growing awakening masses that we need to move from competition, back to cooperation, for the old ways of living together have demonstrably failed. As The Mayan's predicted The Age of Integrity is overcoming the age of Power. This change began on 22nd of December 2012 according to their teachings. Human kind will ascend to Community or Common-Unity. The meek shall inherit the earth, hey?

"My Connection to Source!"

Many times, throughout the day, without moving my head, I cast my gaze upward and to the right and wink at the universe, just to remind him that I AM watching him for he is a trickster and has a wicked sense of humour. I do this just to keep him on track and doing the work that I commanded, which is to fulfil my conscious life intention:" I AM here to have a gentle, joyful, loving, healthy and abundant life", that is my command. Since I put that in place, that is precisely how my life is unfolding, I don't have to DO anything, just BE. It IS working for me. So I see the universe as friend, companion and servant and I often giggle at the tricks he plays.

"Beyond Codependency".

G'day folks, after making great progress in healing my childhood wounds I then embarked on a journey to DE-program myself from co- dependent behaviour.

So in about 1995 I began. For me this behaviour is best understood by listening to any love song"My life is empty with out you babe" and others of that ilk. It was a belief that someone else could complete me, that my life would be fantastic if I had someone in my life that could fill the holes in my soul.

This little phrase steered me out of my co-dependent behaviour:"Unsolicited advice is abuse" and I'll tell you why. In my journey, when I AM struggling the most, that is when I learn the most. Unfortunately, when I appear to be struggling, that's when all the rescuers show up, with phrases like"I know what you need to do mate" This remark and others like it are all useless, for I AM the only one that can ever know what my needs are, how can it be otherwise? So when someone says that to me I usually reply with"Sorry mate, but I AM here to live my life my way, not your way, if you want to be a true friend then be around when I put up my hand and ask for help, I respect your sovereignty, I expect the same in return.

Another phrase that I found useful was"All opinions are worthless", for when I share my story with you, or my truth, if you like, and you reply with your opinion of my truth, it has no value for me. It won't change my truth, only I can do that, and tells me nothing about you and your truth, so for me"opinions are like hearsay evidence in court" totally in-valid, the only thing that has any merit is personal life experience or witnessed testimony. All this, for me, Is related to"The Power of I AM", and there is plenty of stuff out there on that topic. So, this is how I moved through step 2 on my journey to reclaim my authentic self. It worked for me. Frank Sinatra:"I did it MY WAY"! Haha.

"Men In Pain".

Why?

For me the reason men are in so much pain is because for centuries they have been denied access to their own most powerful healing tool,"Feelings"!

"Big Boys don't cry, Suck it up, Deal with it, If you don't stop crying I will give you something to cry for, Man-up, just a few hammers that come to mind.

In my own journey,I spent over 20 years trying to think my way out of depression and it only got worse, It was not until I learned how to silence my mind, that I could hear my heart, and so I started feeling the pain of depression and allowing those feelings that had been locked inside me to fully express. For me, Depression was a gift for it drove me to find my own soul-utions.

So now, I listen to my heart and body and obey them, whatever feelings come up I express them in the moment (depending on location, haha) and allow them to discharge. Depression was just a spiritual wake up call, a rite of passage and a natural human response to having to live in such a corrupt and oppressive society!

"Feelings are Healings"!

"Being vulnerable is just a human being, BEING HUMAN!" "Master and Commander":

In 2004 I got my Master 5 marine qualification and I became a skipper in the Whitsunday Islands.

I remember the first time I took a boat out. It suddenly dawned on me,"Bugga Bob, You are totally responsible for the lives of all these people, the safety of the vessel and crew even the energy on this cruise". Talk about a wake up Call. I had recently watched that movie"Master and Commander", so all I did was to take that ideology and apply it to my own life.

I AM "Master and Commander" of my life and I take full responsibility for this life that I do create. Every event that happens in my life holds a lesson for me, i just have to find and learn it.

So being"Master and Commander" I asked my self,"What is my life purpose?", so I set my life purpose to be:"To simply find my own truth". Bang, I got the big one out of the way, next, as a spiritual being having a human experience,"How do I want to experience this life?; so I set my conscious life intention to be:"I AM here to have a gentle, joyful, loving, healthy and abundant life" and that is how my life is unfolding.

The "here to have part is my direct command to the universe to provide what I have commanded, but it is also my address, so the universe knows where to deliver it.

Since I put that intention in place I AM just cruising, for the universe is doing all the hard work and I have no fear of the future for I know it will align with my intention. It is working for me.

"The Letter to Mum".

Dear Mum, I am writing to you to tell you how it felt for me growing up in our family. This is not about blame, just telling you my story, look forward to hearing yours, your loving son Bob.

And so I sat down and wrote and wrote about how I hated being hit so often or how she never came to school sports days, how she kept reminding me of the scar on her belly, any way. what I thought would be one or two pages turned into another WAR and PEACE but at least I got it all out. I posted this epic to Mum back in the UK and that was the hardest thing I had ever done, but I knew it was the way forward for I was being torn apart by" I hate my Mum for what She did to me, but you have to love your MUM!" this quandary was tearing my soul apart!

Six months later I get a reply, I am so sorry Bobby, you must think I am the worst mother in the world. I replied, no Mum I am just sharing my story, tell me yours! Time passes, a lot of it, then finally a letter from Mum arrives and she shares her story. She was born in 1924 in Germany between the wars her Dad was an alcoholic and her mum was a control freak, her cousins joined the SS or they were shot, it was a pretty horrific childhood and the I realised that Mum was just passing on what had been dumped on her and with that understanding I was able to move from hate back to a place of love, and I felt so much lighter for that. A couple of days later, once I had stopped crying, I phoned Mum in England to learn that she was back in hospital with a second bout of bowel cancer, so

I contacted the hospital and managed to speak to MUM and that was the first time and the last time we spoke as Mother and Son as adult to adult, so with tears at both sides of the pond we talked ! Two days later Mum passed away and I was so glad we had come to a loving closure.

A few days went by and I AM feeling much lighter but there is still a little niggle in my shoulders, still a heaviness there, then BOOM! Dad ya Bastard! So I got out the note pad and wrote a letter to DAD. Dad had died awhile back, not sure where or when, so I put the letter in an envelope and addressed it to DAD in Heaven and burnt it! Feeling much lighter now!

"Equal Sovereigns".

I respect your sovereignty, I expect the same in return, for me: all are equal unique and sovereign, and what is this"WE" business? I can only speak for myself. I do not condone or support co-dependent behaviour.

I only ask for what I want, I never tell anyone what to do, for I have no authority over anyone else, it is my job to meet my needs. I come to this forum simply to share my journey, my truth and the steps I have taken to heal myself of my own childhood abuse, and I have.

I do not sugar coat the truth for that is like masking the truth which is tantamount to hiding the truth which is like lying, and for me it is hiding the truth and lying that is keeping the beast of abuse alive.

"Balance".

"If you have not experienced"bad" how can you know what"good" is? If you do not know what you dislike, how can you know what you like? I feel that this duality is essential for a balanced life. Until you have explored the limits of"good" and"bad" how do you know where to let your own pendulum come to rest, for life is all about"balance", hey?

"Knowing or Knowledge".

I prefer"Knowing" to" Knowledge" .Living in Heart space I have found a place that I call my knowing and my knowing has no words, and through that space I have a connection to a place I call the Universal library of all there is to know, which is where I get my soul-utions. Adam and Eve were kicked out of Paradise for eating from the tree of knowledge which says to me that the pursuit of knowledge is the original sin! . This pursuit of knowledge through science and technology really has not benefited us or the planet! I love this insight:"Thinking is the weapon of mass distraction" and you may quote me on that! Woof!

"WE and You".

Yeah co-dependency is a big one, I found my way through by just using"I" statements and only speaking from my own life experience! These two phrases helped me a lot:"unsolicited advice is abuse" and"All opinions are worthless". As all are equal and all are unique, I do not have anyone's answers, I have just found my own soul-utions which work for me. I believe that is the purpose of the inner journey, which is for all to find their own answers.

My latest realisation is that"All I have is my story, my Truth, and the only person it is valid for is me" I now realise that I have no right to speak for the We or for the YOU, for everyone has their own story! It is OK to speak TO the WE and Too the YOU but not for them, get it?

I believe that the best way for us to help each other is to simply share our stories, and that some of the tools I have picked up along the way will resonate with another! I AM the only expert on my life!

"Not Nice".

for me:" I AM not here to be nice, or kind, I AM here to be HONEST!" Simply to share, from a space of Integrity, My Truth, My Story. If you have an emotional response to the information i AM sharing that is YOUR choice, Your phealings are your responsibility not mine, I have no power over you!

I have found that from this posture, compassion naturally flows! WOOF!

Personal Growth! What is it and what is in it for me? For me:

All are Equal and All are Unique, so everyone's journey will be unique!

Personal Growth is the task of discovering my Authentic self, the person I was born to be. Re-establishing absolute belief in my self, Learning to totally trust my In-Tuition and finally getting to a place of contentment.

This work involved healing the wounds of childhood and abandoning behaviour patterns established at that time that enabled me to survive, but are no longer appropriate as an adult. Next was deprogramming from cultural conditioning and co-dependent behaviour, all the while questioning everything, and building my truth from what resonated with my heart.

So, after 26 years,I AM Content, I like me, Me, myself and I get along real well! I AM living my dream and I know that I created it.

So many people say" I have let go of the past" but are still operating under old programs. I believe the work has to be done and is an essential part of the Awakening process, after all what is the use of running Windows 95 when everyone else is using Windows 10. (probably not the best analogy, but you get the idea)

In our current society everyone has been programmed,more or less, no one has retained their original as born state of Innocence and Inner Knowing,and Reclaiming that is the work of"Personal Growth".

I have no ones answers, my job is to find my own. All I can share is my experience, my story, my truth and that is what I do.

Love and Light. Bob

ps: Personal Growth is not a spectator sport, It IS Personal and it is Growth, so come on in, the water is fine!

"Opinions are Worthless".

for me:"Why all opinions are worthless". After I have shared my truth and someone comes back with their opinion of my truth, for me it has no value. #1 it will not change my truth, only I can can do that and I do for my story is organic. #2 your opinion of my story tells me nothing about you and your truth, only that you have a lot of opinions, and something else I noticed, opinions always come from Headspace and are always a response to a perceived challenge, an ego based knee jerk reaction ! Beyond Codependency and loving it! Woof!

"Teachers?"

ADULTS ONLY!

for me, all are equal and all are unique, and from that platform the concept of anyone being a"Teacher" is unsupportable. All I have is my story, my truth and my own unique skill set,and I know that the only person they are valid for is me. My only hope, by sharing my story,is that some elements may resonate with another equal being, who will enfold them into their own journey, and in that way by sharing our truth all can grow together! Anyone claiming to be a Teacher or a Guru has already invalidated the belief that all are equal! So, be wary of anyone who claims to be a Teacher or A Guru, for all they have is their own story and for them to assume it is valid for any other being is pure arrogance and an entirely egocentric posture! Ruthless in Purity! Woof!

"Labels".

I am not your "fan" for I do not idolise anyone because for me ALL ARE EQUAL! for me a fan is something that spins round and blows a lot of wind. I connect to you because the energy is nurturing for me, and when it is no longer nurturing I will drop it! and as for your penchant for putting labels on people, I do not accept any labels for ALL ARE UNIQUE and the only label that would apply to all is I AM UNIQUE and also by putting labels on people you have made a judgement about them and as ALL ARE EQUAL what right do you have to Judge anyone? The only place for labels in my life is in the supermarket and the Pharmacy so that I can be informed about what I AM ingesting! All I have is my truth and my story and it only applies to me! get my drift? Merry Christmas! Woof!

"Trust".

"Creative Visualisation" I would like everyone to consider this image, just for a moment, if you will: Imagine a world where everyone makes their decisions based on Trust instead of Fear! Just imagine what that world might look like! Picture it for yourselves, what does it pheal like for you? And now that this Intention is out there I will be interested to see where it goes! Woof!

"Contentment".

for me: Contentment does not exist outside of YOU!. It resides deep, deep within You! and it is your job to find it. No one else can find your Contentment for YOU! So, as All-ways the choice, whether conscious or unconscious is YOURS! I AM that I AM and I AM CONTENT! ps: As an afterthought, you might like to substitute the words "authenticity" and "Integrity" for the word "contentment" The rationale is still the same! Woof!

"Noticing".

Simply Noticing all these amazing intellects racing around in "Headspace" looking for answers to this current mess, and only finding more questions, for there are NO answers in "Headspace" and so the Hamster wheel keeps turning as it has done for thousands of years! For me, the only "Soulution" resides in "Heartspace" in that inner silence wherein dwells certainty, contentment and Knowing! woof!

"So Many, So Few"

So many hearing: so few listening, So many thinking: so few phealing, So many judging: so few accepting, So many denying: so few validating, SAD hey?

"Nature's Way"

For most of my adult life I have held a close connection to the ocean, the sea and to natures way!

I have travelled this world and connected to many different races, colours and creeds, and in those quiet times in the desert and in the midst of oceans I have connected with other species.

I have yet to meet up with a transvestite dolphin or a homosexual whale, for all that I notice when I look at other species, they are all gainfully employed in meeting their prime directive; the survival of their own species. It is only in Man that I see a corruption of Nature's Way, an almost manic joy in celebrating traits that will only lead to it's own demise. For me, I know where I stand. I stand with both bare-feet firmly planted on Nature's Way!

"Lost the plot!" by Barnaby.

I do so love Dad's "Lost the Plot" days. We have so much Fun. Our day began at 05:30 ish, whatever that is with skinny dipping around the boat as the sun rose over Mandalay Point, then back on board to dance naked on the deck to the sounds of the"Battlefield Band" at full bore until we were dry. Then down below for brekkie and a cuddle before we rowed ashore. Well Dad rowed I AM Navigator! Did some fiction stuff and a few essentials like fresh roo mince and bikkies for me and tobacco and rum and steak for dad, then a romp on the beach where I chased shadows and dad did rolly polly's until it was time to head home. Dad started the Tohatsu, bless you (always sounds like a sneeze to me) and we cruised eastward across the bay pounding into the surf. It was at this point that Dad broke out into our"ring ting clang clang woof woof" song. I love this one and you can use the words to any tune you know! Try it! Back on board with a full belly and sore ribs from giggling so much, Ah Bliss! Oh,sorry, how rude of me! how was your day! Woof!

"A World Turned Upside Down".

My Heartfelt thanks to Leon Rosselson, a fellow Folksinger turned writer, for the inspiration for this following message:

For many months now, I have been pondering the value system of our current society, just looking at what"WE" hold in highest esteem, and what follows is my own assessment.

#1 Actors.

Actors are placed at the highest level of our society, they are worshipped, mimicked and held high and applauded, but what for? For never showing their true selves, for living a fiction. What do they produce, and can you eat it?

#2 Sportsmen.

They get paid millions for putting a ball in the ground, or through a hoop, or crossing the line first, but what do they produce, can you eat it? Just like actors, they only feed the couch potatoes, hey?

#3 Politicians.

A strange breed of humans, that are supposed to enact the will of the people, yet all they do is line their own pockets, at the expense of our innate Freedoms ! A breed of parasites that do not benefit humanity,

#4 Just a bucket for all the other parasites on our ascension.

Folks like Gurus, and Psychologists, and Psychiatrists and Motivational Speakers and 25 year old "Life Coaches" who must be fraud, hey? How can they claim to be a life coach when they are only, at best, one third of the way through their own lives? For thousands of years people have got their guidance from the wisdom of their own tribal elders.

So, where are our elders now, and how are they treated ? Locked up in age care prisons, doped up to the eyeballs with anti-depressants and fed on swill!

"Meekness".

What this covid fallacy has shown me, is what, or who, is important, so here and now I express my thanks, to the ordinary people, like farmers, and truck drivers, and nurses, and everyone else who is engaged in selfless support of their neighbours.

"And the meek shall inherit the earth", but, never mistake my meekness, for weakness . YOU HAVE BEEN WARNED!

"The five stages of Healing".

For me: I went through five stages to heal from my own childhood abuse.

1, INNOCENCE,

This stage began when I was born as a magical innocent being, and the world was a wondrous place. This lasted for less than two years when, through abuse I moved into stage two.

2, VICTIM-HOOD,

as a small child I was unable to defend myself and became a victim of my violent surroundings. This stage lasted until I was about 12 or 13 and was able to say NO and defend myself.

3, SURVIVOR,

and so I started maturing as a survivor, using the fight or flight behaviours I had developed as a victim, like being perfect, being the people pleaser, believing what"adults" told me. This stage lasted until I was 32 years old and had my first"panic attack", and began my dance with depression. Although it did not feel like it then,this marked my shift into stage 4.

4, RECOVERY,

1984 was the beginning of my recovery. Unfortunately, I wasted about 20 years trying to think my way out of depression. I have an amazing intellect, but it did not help me solve my problems. Looking back I call this"The Trap of the Intellect". In 1992 I came across John Bradshaw's work on the inner child and so I began healing the wounds of my childhood, deprogramming myself from co-dependent behaviour, and re-establishing my belief in Me. At this time I had been taking various anti-depressants for about 10 years, with another 10 years to go. In 2005 when I became a ships captain I decided to take full responsibility for my life and look at this pain I was feeling. This was a pivotal time for me, when I realised that the pain I was feeling was just a natural human response to living in such a un- human society and because I was living the life that was expected of me, I was not living my truth, and so I began the mission to find my own truth, and walk my own talk. I could not think my way out, so I tried to FEEL my way out and that was my pathway out of depression, it was through feeling all the pain of my childhood, and releasing all those trapped feelings, that I finally healed, and threw away all medications and started listening to my heart, obeying my body, and totally trusting my Inner-Tuition. This finally brought me to stage 5.

5, CONTENTMENT.

Now, I AM content with me. I have found my truth and I know it is my truth, for it resonates with my heart, and I totally trust my Inner- Tuition. My life now is so simple, for I live in Heartspace not Headspace, and my life is unfolding just as I have directed it to. My life is awesome, for I create it that way!

SUMMARY:

I spent about 2 years in Innocence, then 10 years as a Victim, moving to about 20 years as a Survivor and nearly 30 years in Recovery, and finally being content with me for the last 8 years. It's been a long and challenging road, but I AM glad I did the work of self discovery.

I AM Master and Commander of my life, and I DO take full responsibility for this life that I create, and if I can do it, so can others, hey?

For me, all are SUE: Sovereign, Unique and Equal, and the universe operates under the KISS principle, Keep It Simple, Sovereign. Life is supposed to be simple, hey?

Personal Insights

I love this one:" I had to go out of my mind, to come to my senses". I experience this life through my senses, I feel the warmth of the sun on my skin, I smell the sweet tang of the rotting mangoes, I hear the song of the birds, I feel the texture of the ground beneath my bare feet, so I FEEL my life, I do not THINK it, ergo: I FEEL therefore I AM.

"Bliss is momentary, Contentment is Eternal".

"It is more important to open your heart, than open your mind".

I always and all-ways listen to my body. When my body is tired, WE sleep, and when my body is awake, WE play! I experience this life through my senses, I feel the warmth of the sun on my skin, I hear the sound of the birds in the trees, I smell the sweet tang of the rotting mangoes and I taste the bitterness of my coffee, so"I had to go out of my mind, to come to my senses". Descarte's was wrong, hey?:

"In the silence of my heart, I have found a place I call my Knowing, and my Knowing has no words".

"Whatever is not nurturing for me, I simply call the beast, and I no longer feed the beast".

"Depression is not an illness, but a natural response to living in slavery".

"Until you can silence your mind, you will never have, Peace of mind"

"My heart is my only compass, and my Inner-tuition, my only guide". " Thinking is the weapon of mass distraction".

"If you live in fear, your fears will engulf you". "Phealings are Healings".

"The Feelings you swallow may one day choke you".

"Sometimes I AM happy, sometimes I AM sad, but I AM always content for I create my life".

"My mind is just a tool that I use when I choose, for I AM so much more than my mind".

" My words are my spells, so I do cast them wisely, for the universe is always listening and takes everything I say,literally, Literally!"."

" I FEEL, therefore I AM".

"My boundaries are the golden frame around the masterpiece that is me".

"Within the wholeness of creation I see myself as a raindrop in the ocean. I AM aware of the ebb and flow of creation, but I still know the raindrop that is me".

"It is my job to complete me".

" There are no gurus, there are no experts, as all are equal and unique, everyone is only sharing what works for them. To assume that it works for another is just arrogance".

" I AM the only expert on my life!".

If you are thinking about your Intuition, you are in the wrong place"!

"Whether you believe you can, or you believe you can't, you will always be right".

"Religion is for those folks that are afraid of going to hell, Spirituality is for those folks that have already been there!"

Child abuse:"Persecuting the perpetrators is not the answer, for it feels like home to them,for they still feel persecuted. Hurt People, Hurt, People! the only way forward is to help them to heal their own wounds!"

"If you have not experienced"bad" how can you know what"good" is? If you do not know what you dislike, how can you know what you like? I feel that this duality is essential for a balanced life. Until you have explored the limits of"good" and"bad" how do you know where to let your own pendulum come to rest, for life is all about"balance", hey?

It is the arrogance of the scientific community that is destroying our planet. To think they can improve on Nature. I fully support technologies that work with nature. When ever they synthesise something from nature they never capture the whole benefit of the plant or substance, just one little part of it. For me: Science is the sickness and Nature is the cure!

It is not our age that defines our maturity, but our behaviour.

Every day I plant a little seed that will blossom,and bring me joy in my new tomorrow.

there comes a time during a hug when both hearts synchronise, that's called entrainment and that is when the true hug begins

My most important friendship is my friendship with me!

"If all you want to do is to fit in, you never will, for you are unique, so get used to it!"

" If you do not believe in yourself, no-one else will, hey?"

"What once were my demons, are now butterflies in my garden".

The sheep are so terrified of the wolf they do not realise that it is the shepherd that will be eating them, hey?

The most potent vaccine you will ever need, resides within the God given gift of your own immune system. What saddens me at this time is, so many people trust science and technology more than they trust creation! So to all those that believe that science will save them, enjoy your life in cognitive dissonance, it will be a sad and fearful one, I believe in the power of creation, who is with me?

When I had my first panic attack in November 1984. It wasn't my mind that was disturbed it was my body. It took 20 years for me to realise that I could not think my way out I had to listen to my body, and I did.

"Not every door will open, only those that will serve you".

What I find very interesting is that currently there are so many people fighting against the chaos and and fear out there in the world today, but they don't realise that what is going on"out there" is merely a reflection of their own"Inner World"."Heal Yourself, Heal the Planer", hey?

There is no Out there, Out there, and if you are not creating your life, WHO is? pun intended.

Once upon a time, I too had"triggers", until I realised that my triggers were showing me what I needed to work on, so I did the work. I no longer condone or support codependent behaviour, and for me : Political correctness is the epitome of codependency and the antithesis of free speech. So, now,,I continue to spontaneously share my heart centered truth, and if you have a problem with that, then it is your problem not mine. Avaniceday!

My Heart is my only compass, and my Inner-Tuition is my only guide. I AM the only expert on my life, hey?

On a global scale, there are only two games being played: #1,"Divide and Conquer", so, anyone that is pointing the finger at something, or someone else, for the pain in their lives, is playing that game. #2,"Unite and Thrive", for we are all in this together, and Hurt People Hurt people, but hurt people do not deserve punishment, they deserve our compassion and support in healing their own wounds."Suffer all the little children to come unto me" notice he said all and not"only those that have not been abusers". In my own journey it was not untill I could forgive my abusers, that my healing was complete. If you are not taking responsibility for your life, then you are victim by default, hey?

It's funny how"The bigger the lie" the more it is believed, and the bigger the truth, the more it is denied, strange hey?

I AM not here to be popular, I AM here to be REAL!

It is not the right answers that you are looking for, but the right questions, hey?

"Smart phone, Dumb people, maybe if commonsense was an app, more folks would use it" ?

"Why are you all so afraid of losing the plot, when you never had one to begin with?"

Ha, If it was not true it might be funny, The church in brackets. is the second most powerful financial institution on the planet. They have been robbing us for millennia to saturate their coffers, and yet somewhere in the scriptures I recall that Jesus cast out the usurers and money lenders from the temple . Jesus is a construct, We are all divine, I do not need to pay to join someones club to convene with my Higher Power. I am, We are all Whole ly, holy? For all, that stay centred and aligned with human principles that surely predate Christianity, like Integrity, Intuition, empathy, why bow down to this charade? And if there is a God!, Why is he always short of Money?

I have no problem speaking too the WE, or too the YOU, but I can never speak for the WE, or for the YOU.

"The Feelings that you have swallowed, WILL, one day come back and choke you", hey?

"If you don't speak your truth, you will never live it", hey?

There is NO-Thing out there, that has any power over me, for I take full responsibility for this life that I DO create.

"Passion comes from the Heart, Not the Mind", hey? How can we rise up if we keep putting each other down?

for me: Feeling alone is a natural and essential aspect of leadership, just ask any ship's captain. To be able to stand calmly in my own heart centered truth and make the decisions I have to make to bring my ship and crew back home safely Is just part of my job, so if you are uncomfortable within standing alone in your own truth, you will never be a leader, for you are still seeking approval from others, and that is just co-dependent behaviour, hey? So to all you folks that are still hiding behind WE, YOU or US, when are you going to share your own truth? and take full responsibility for your life? and stop enticing others into your own victim-hood?

By finding my own truth, I have removed fear from my life! "There are No rabbit holes in Heartspace".

"Living in the NOW, the concept of Time, is irrelevant", hey?

"In the NOW, and without rhyme or reason, or any need for justification, everything just"IS". Eckhart Tolle' refers to this as the Is-ness of all things, and I get that, do you?

"Humanity is insane, Peace costs nothing, but War makes beggars of us all"!

I view the universe as a huge jigsaw puzzle, and everyone holds one piece. As each person heals themselves they colour in their own piece of this puzzle, and so the broader picture becomes clearer for us all, hey?

for me:" Pills, Promote Illness & Long Lasting Servitude", hey?

I know I AM Knocking on a bit, but at 68 I AM going great, and at this stage of my life, I would rather BE LOVE, than make love, especially up here in the tropics, too much like hard work, hey? So here is to Being Love! YAY!"KISS".

History is just His, Story, it does not mean it is the truth. The truth is something you have to discern for yourself, hey?

I AM not insane, this society IS! YAY. Integrity:

Such a simple word, but in this age of ascension, the most powerful word in the world! Our lift into the age of Integrity, began on the 21st of December 2012, according to the Mayans. It will take awhile for the age of Integrity to eclipse the outgoing age of power, but it is happening, just look around the world, more and more folks are finding their own truth, and the courage to speak it, so, if you are not comfortable in speaking your truth because you might offend someone, well good luck with that! Those not standing in their own Integrity, will be left behind. Mark my words, YOU have been warned. See you on the other side, hey?

"A Piece of Paper".

My Sovereignty, my Freedoms, do not depend on the existence or non existence of some piece of paper, for they are my birthright and cannot be taken away. Only I, can give them away, hey?

"Cognitive Dissonance".

Here is a prime example: If anti depressants were effective, the suicide rate should be falling, but it is not, it is increasing, just as much as the sales of anti depressants are. This says to me, being a simple bloke, that anti depressants are killing people, just as they were intended to. AM I the only one making this connection? So while you are all busy trying to grow carrots holistically, what's the point, when there will be no one left to tend your gardens? What are your priorities?

Out There.

"Nothing, Out There, has any impact on the contentment I get from living in Heartspace".

Entertainment.

for me, the search for knowledge is very entertaining for the mind but not essential for growth. I prefer the KNowing of Heartspace to the Knowledge of Headspace, hey?

SUE

for me: All are SUE, Sovereign, Unique and Equal, therefore it follows that, as I AM unique, I AM the only one in the whole of creation that can ever know what my needs are, hey? so please stop wasting your time, and more importantly MY time telling me what I need to do or where my duty lies.

BEING.

Within my own BEING, I have a hierarchy: Spirit, Body, Mind, and in that order.

Embracing Nature.

My intention for this message is to spark a response from everyone here, about how they, on a daily basis bring more of Nature into their own lives.

This is what I AM up to at the moment:

#1 I walk this land barefoot, I do not own a pair of shoes.

#2 I spend as much time as I can out in Nature, skinny dipping in the ocean and dancing naked in the rain.

#3 Consciously removing any toxins I may be exposed to. the biggest of which was my TV or Terror Vision. I have not had a TV since 1995.

#4 I only use rainwater for even bottled water is toxic. Water is a very powerful solvent, hey?

#5 Constantly observing Nature and how she works, and adopting her gifts freely into my life.

#6 I do not use any pharmaceuticals.

There are many more aspects of nature that I work with. For Me: Science is the Sickness, and Nature is the Cure, hey?

So, what are you bringing into your life? please share, for you may have found something that I have missed, hey? Injoy, Bob.

"Beyond Codependency".

"What other people are DOING is none of my bloody business", hey? So I waste no time considering their journey, I just trust that they are doing their very best, as indeed, I AM!

My Knowing.

Within the silence of my heart, I have found a place I call my knowing, and my Knowing has no words, and in that place of knowing, I have created a page called Contentment. On that page I have created a floating mural of all images that portray contentment for me, and these images keep moving like the letters in a pot of alphabet soup. I have used images that hold the feeling of contentment because I have no better way sharing feelings, at the moment! How does one write a feeling, hey?

"My Body is Smarter Than Me".

Back in 1984, when I had my first panic attack, I woke up at 3 am with my arms and legs flailing around and my body doing what ever it wanted too.

If only I had realised then that my body was giving me a message, but I was so afraid of the power of the feelings I was having that I chose not to listen, but instead I went to my doctor for the answers, and ended up numbing down the power of those feelings with anti-depressants. It took me over 20 years to realise that the power of my feelings was not something to be afraid of, for they were just a measure of how powerful I truly AM. So by embracing those feelings I regained my authentic self and became, once again the powerful "I AM". Now, I listen too and obey my body for it knows intuitively what it needs and never hesitates in telling me. If there is pain in my body I know that I need to look at and find the cause and take natural steps to heal that pain, instead of ingesting more toxins like pain killers, I was crazy like that for many years, hahaha,

"Wound of the Soul"

How can you defeat your enemy if you don't know it's true name. For about 130 years we have been told the name of this enemy is"Mental Illness", when in fact it's true name is"Wound of the Soul", which is why no psychologist or psychiatrist has ever cured anyone, for they only work with the mind. Now that we have the true name we can use appropriate tools to eradicate this condition. Healing through Feeling is one of the tools that I used. My mission is to put an end to all suicides, for I know in my heart of hearts that this IS doable!

"Insight Posters"

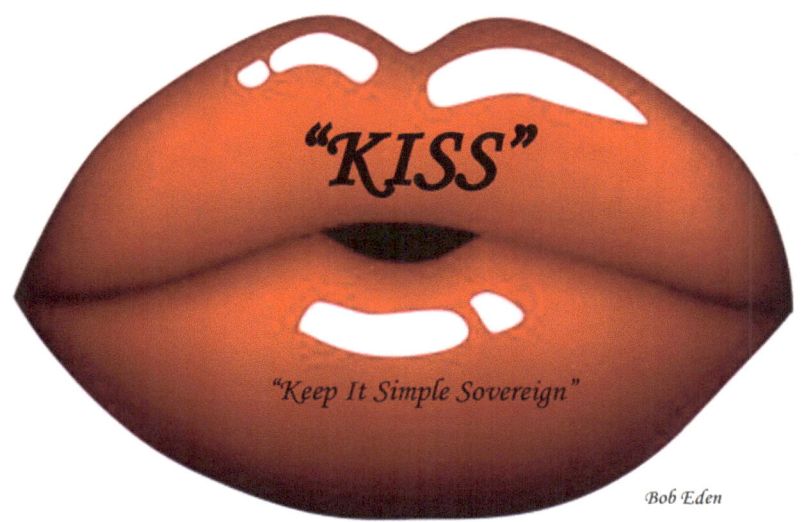

"KISS

"Keep It Simple Sovereign"

Bob Eden

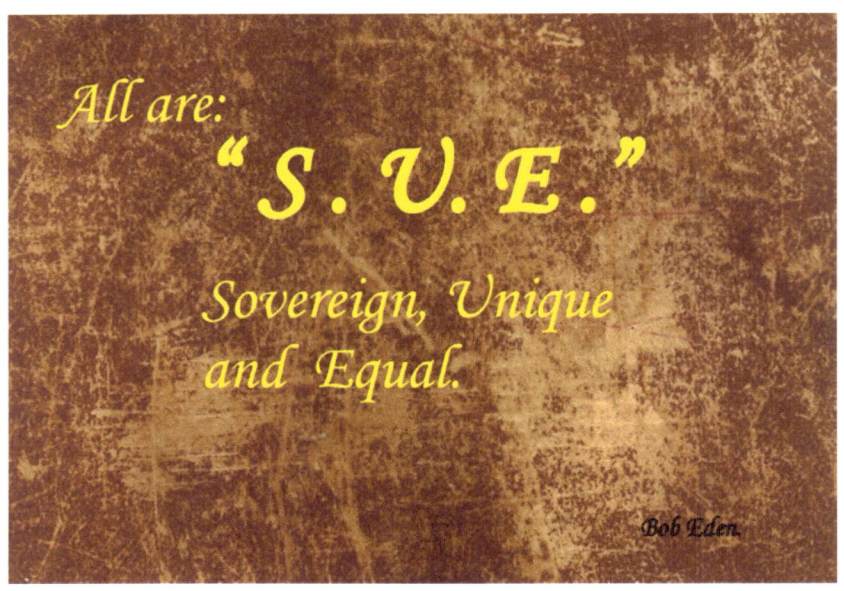

"I AM Master and Commander of My Life".

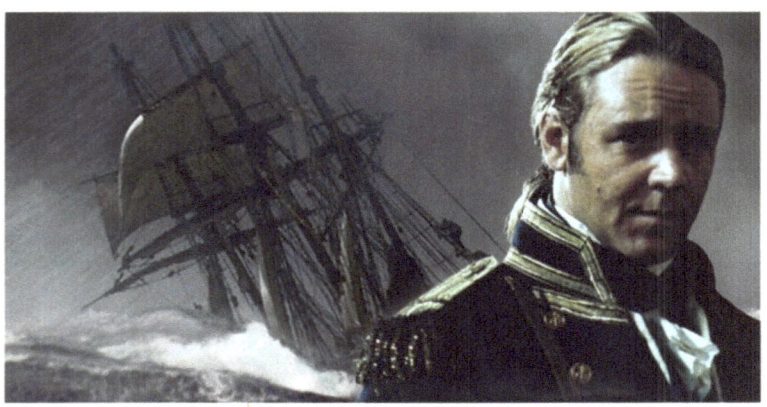

Bob Eden

And I take full responsibility for this life that I DO create!

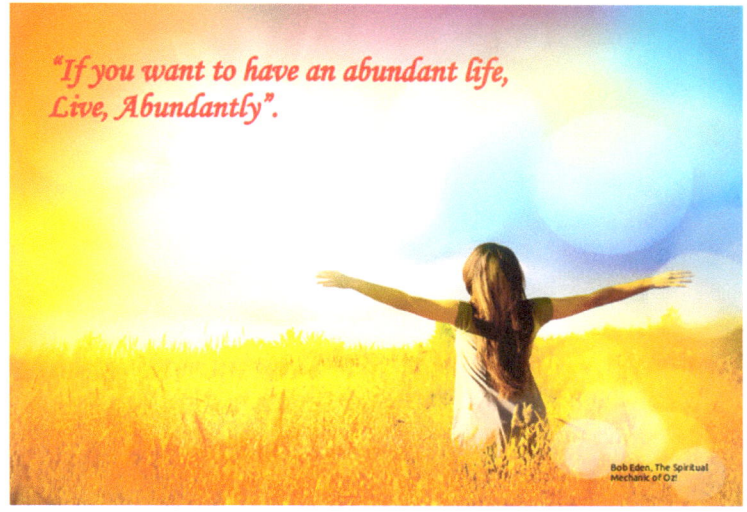

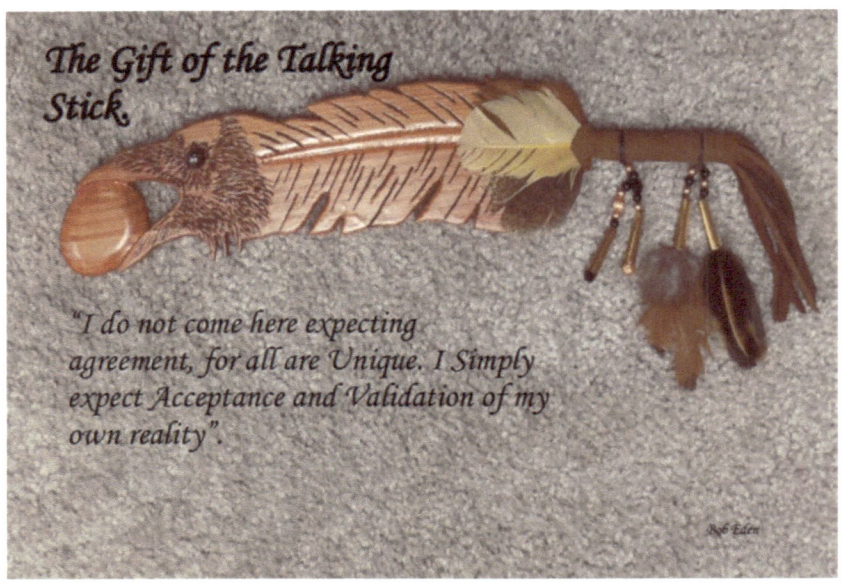

The Gift of the Talking Stick.

"I do not come here expecting agreement, for all are Unique. I Simply expect Acceptance and Validation of my own reality".

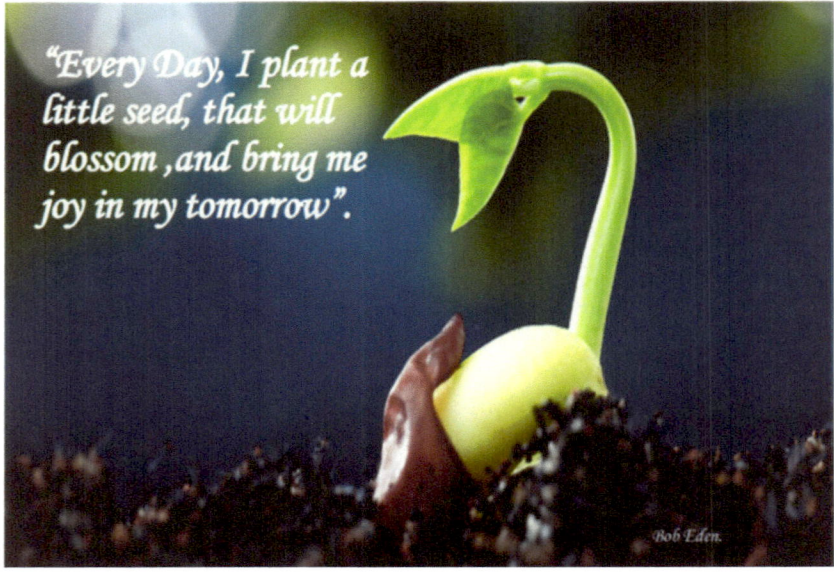

"Every Day, I plant a little seed, that will blossom ,and bring me joy in my tomorrow".

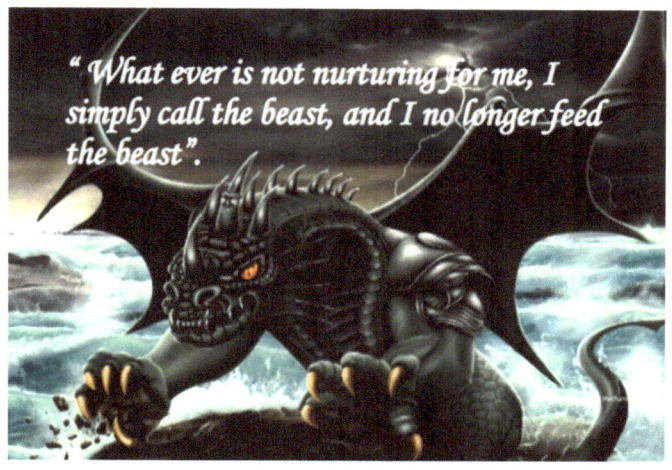

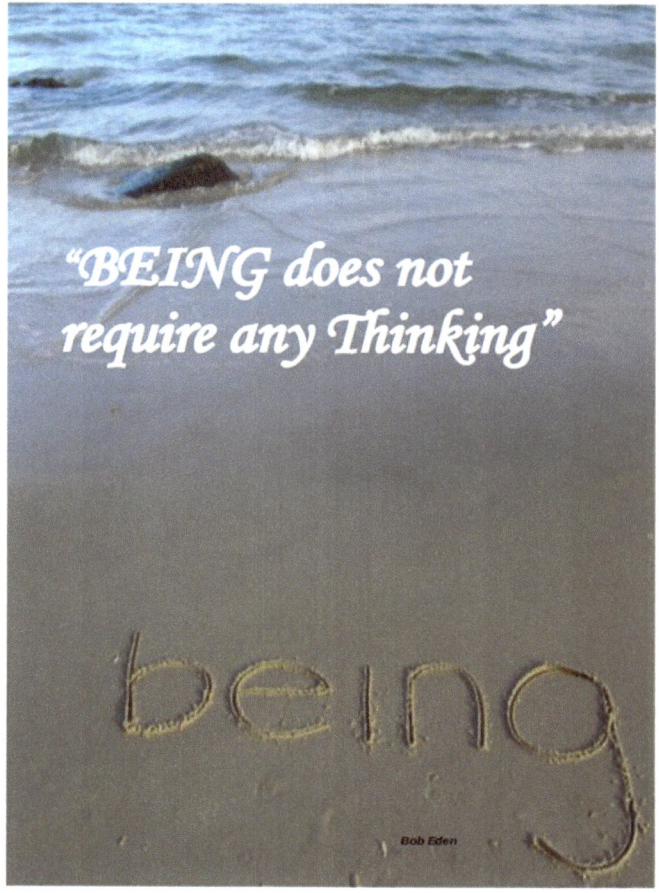

Or Doing, hey?

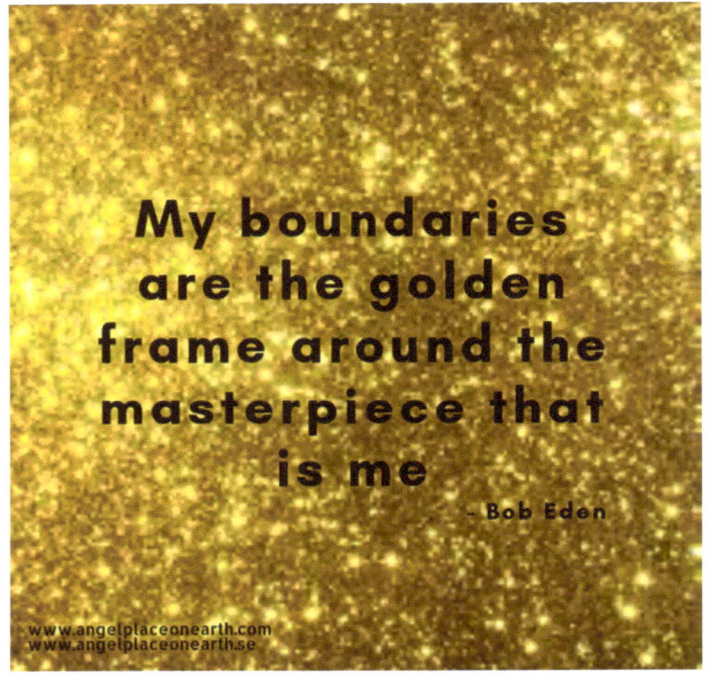

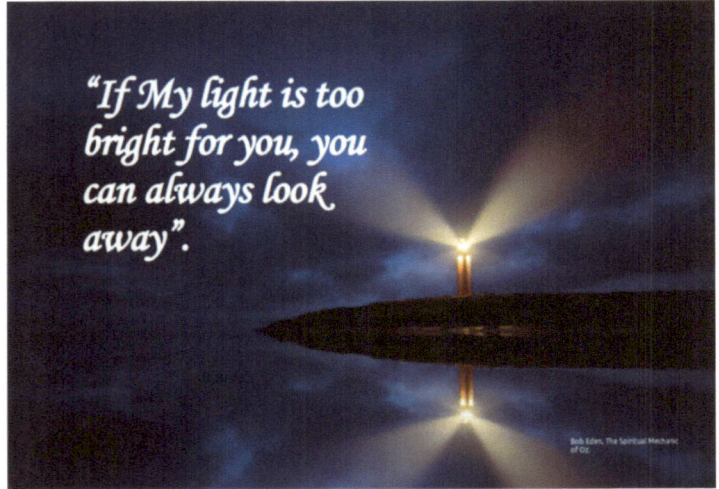

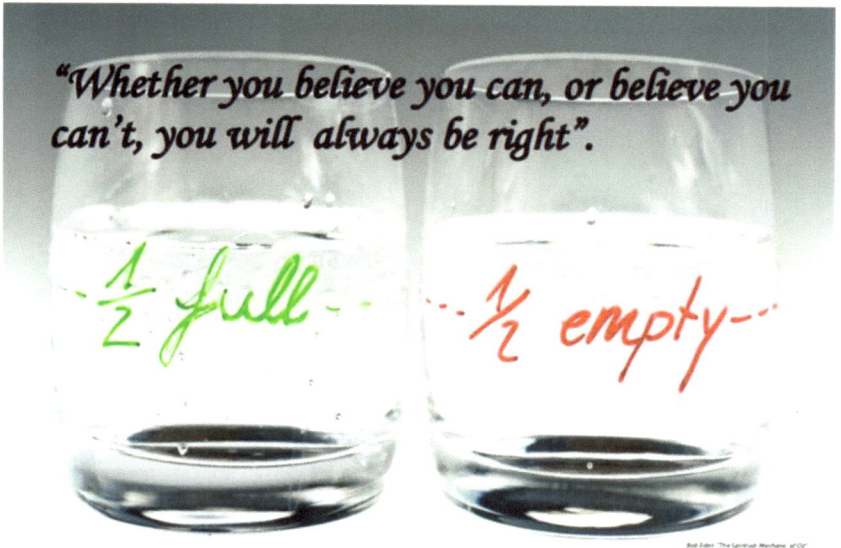

"*Whether you believe you can, or believe you can't, you will always be right*".

½ full · · · ½ empty

"A child that's being abused by its parents doesn't stop loving its parents, it stops loving itself."

~Shahida Arabi
PsychAlive.org

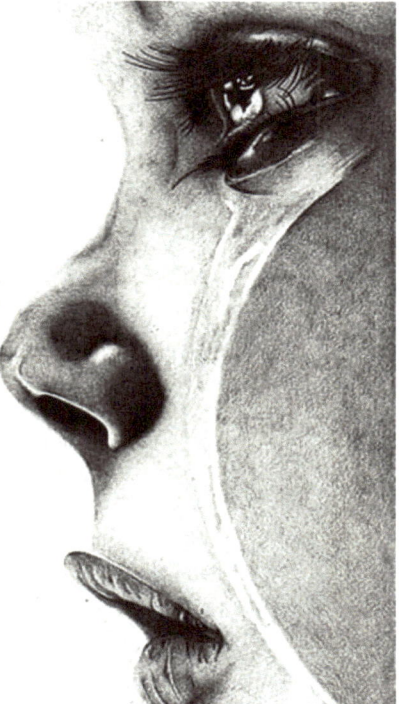

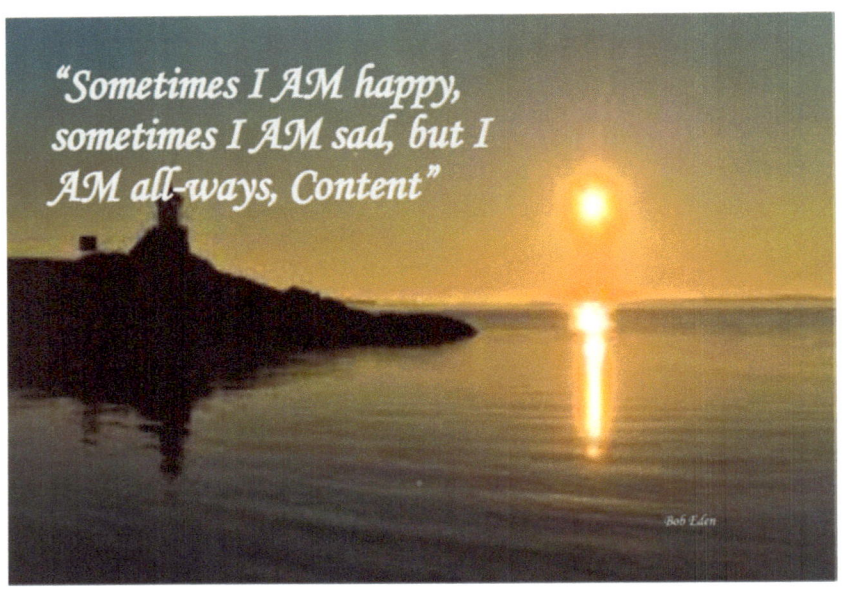

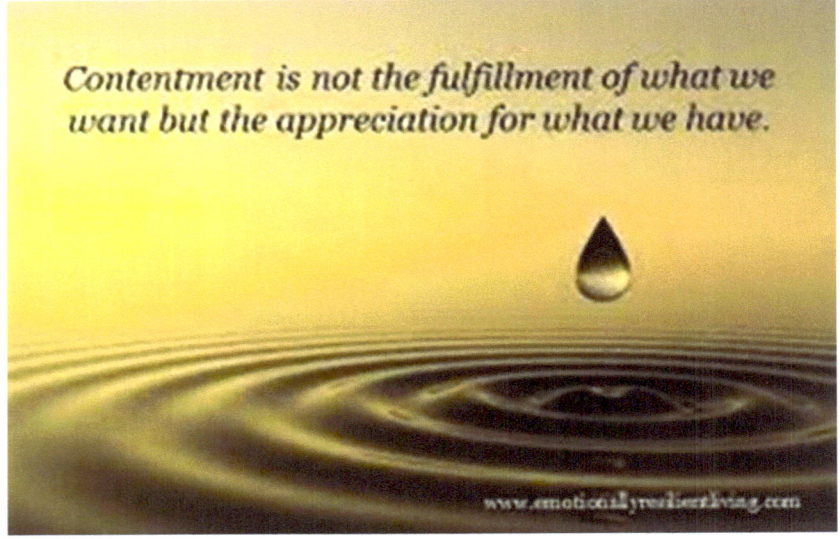

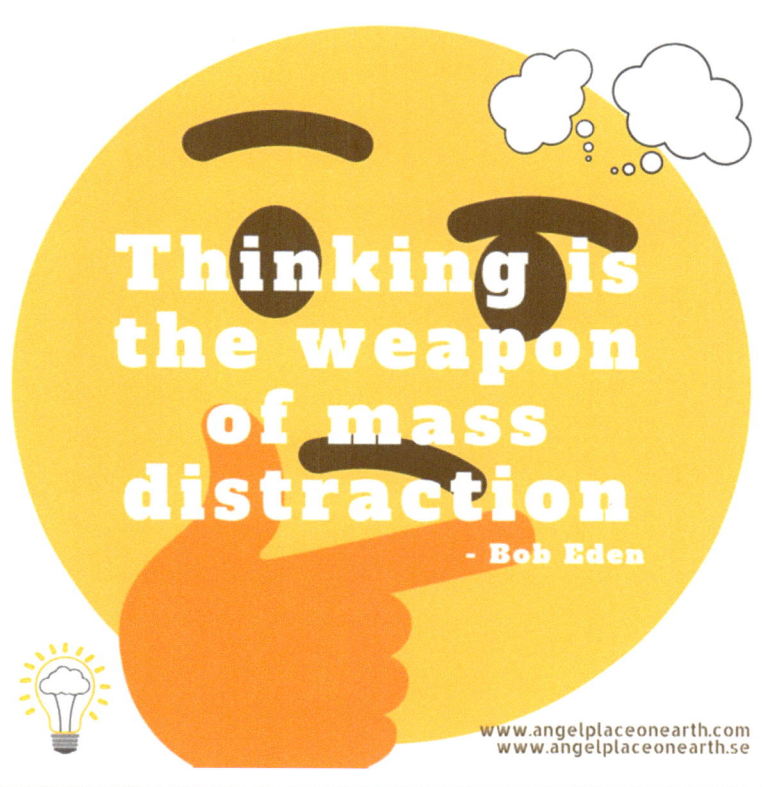

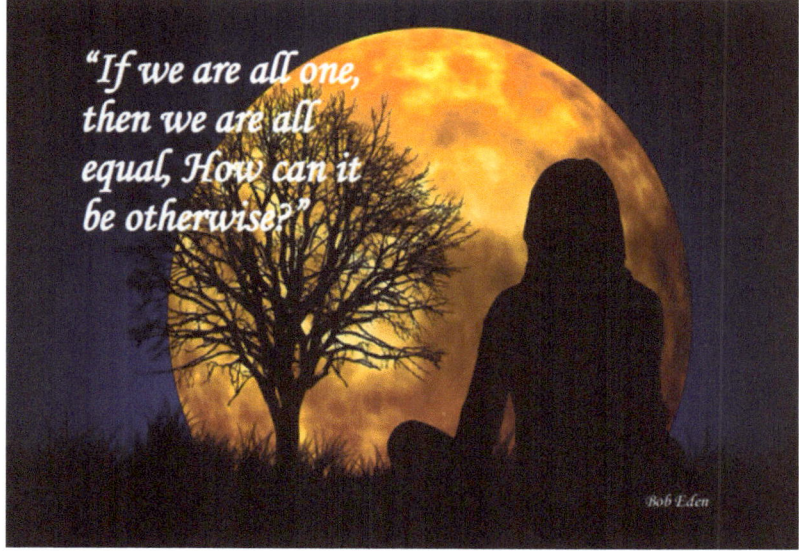

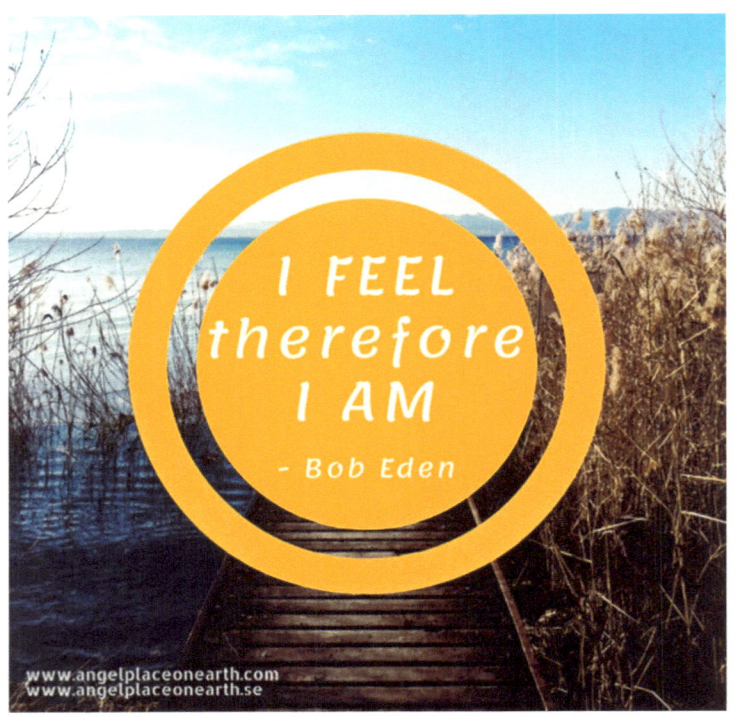

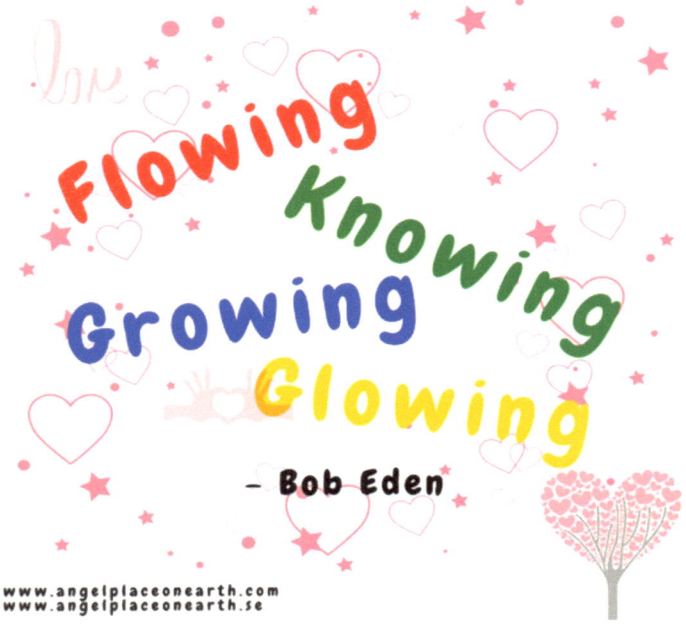

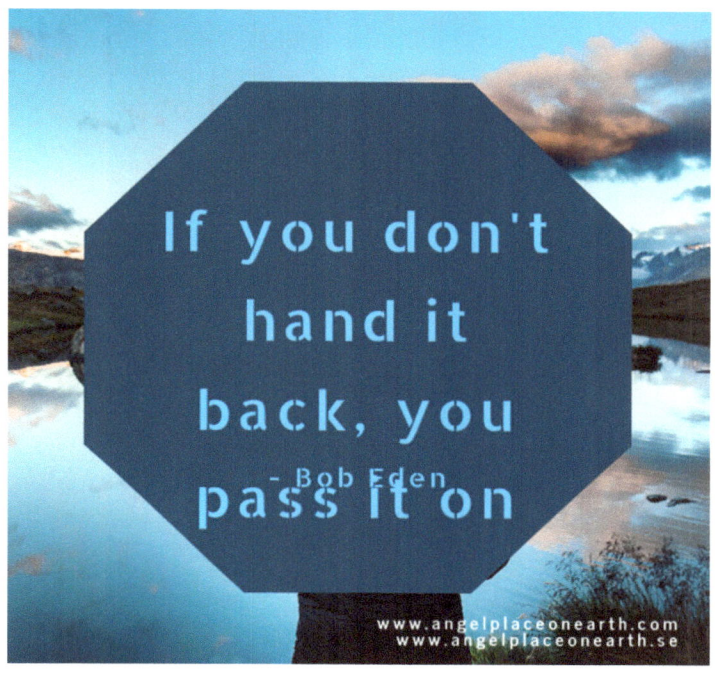

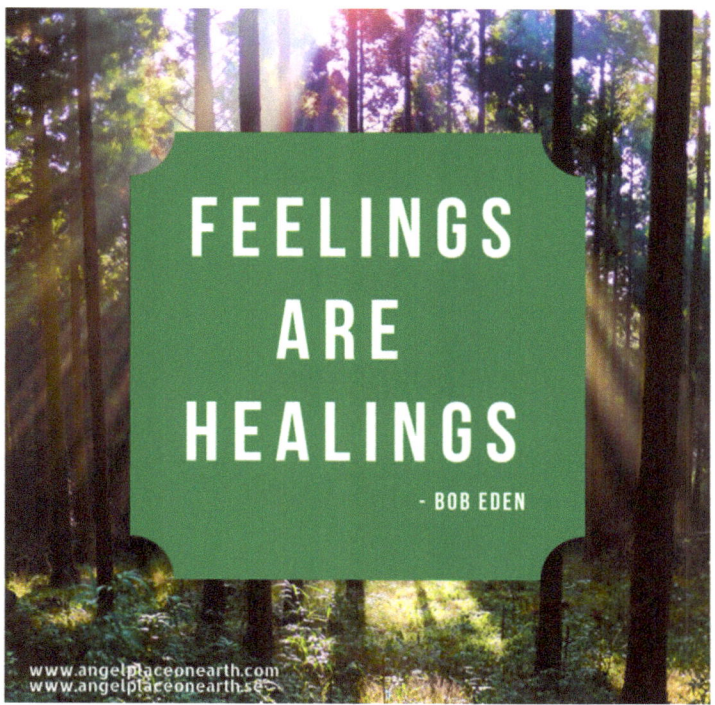

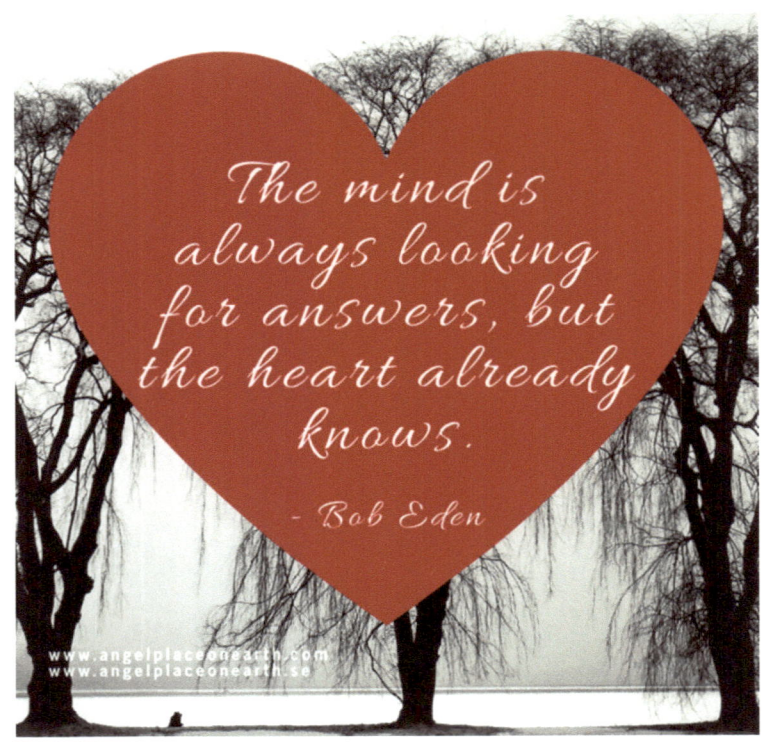

The mind is always looking for answers, but the heart already knows.

- Bob Eden

www.angelplaceonearth.com
www.angelplaceonearth.se

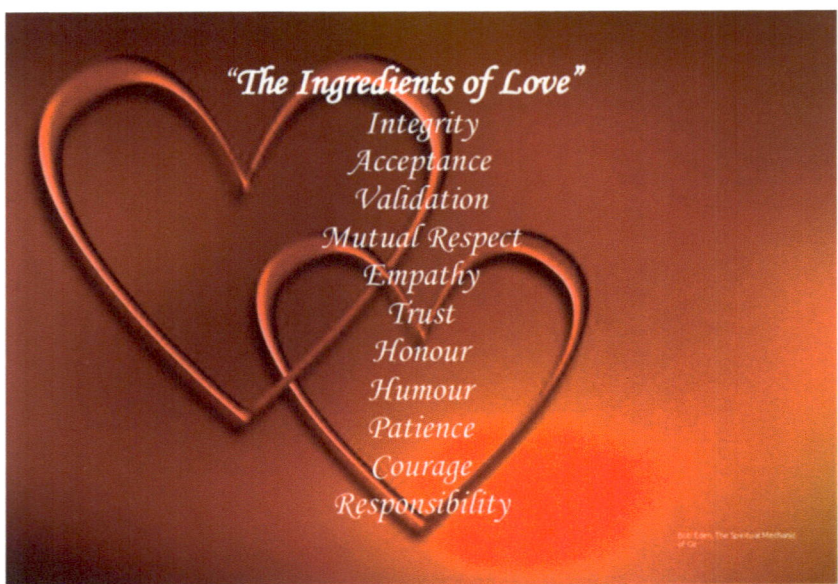

"The Ingredients of Love"

Integrity
Acceptance
Validation
Mutual Respect
Empathy
Trust
Honour
Humour
Patience
Courage
Responsibility

Bob Eden, The Spiritual Mechanic of Oz

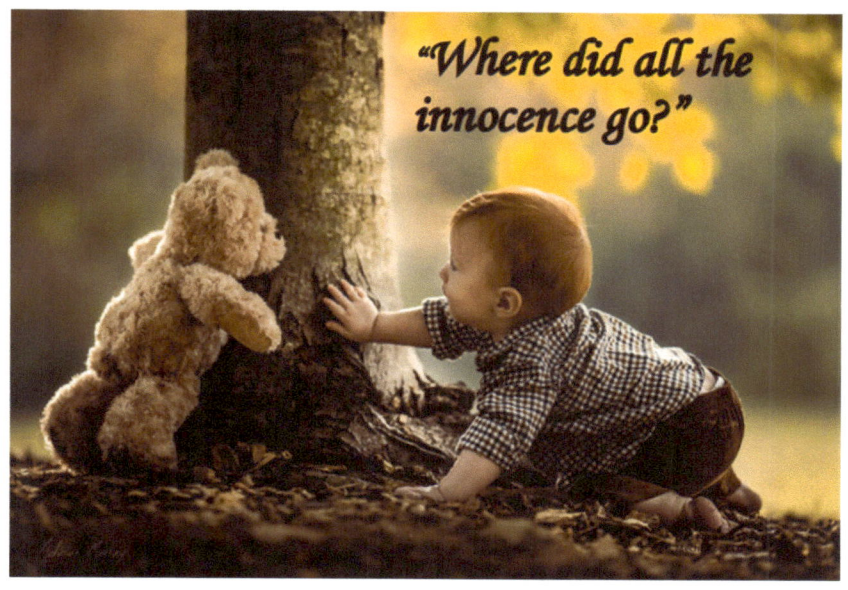

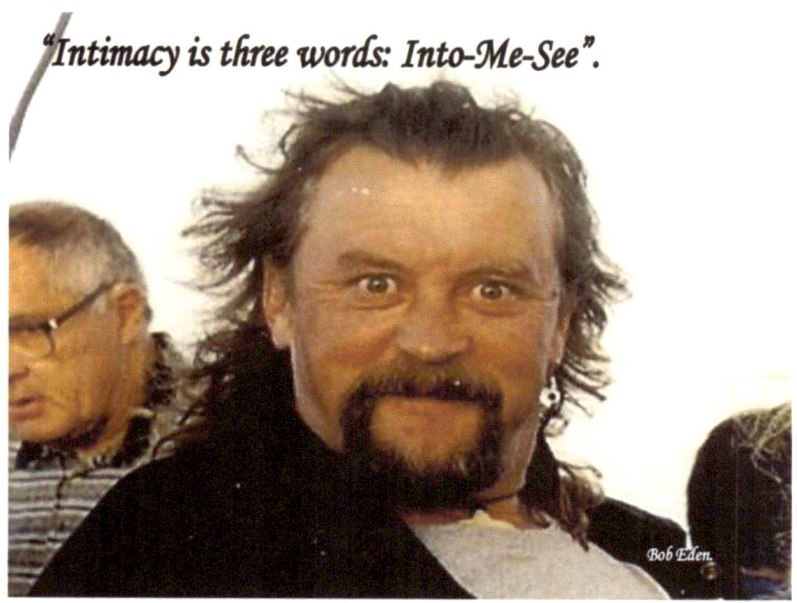

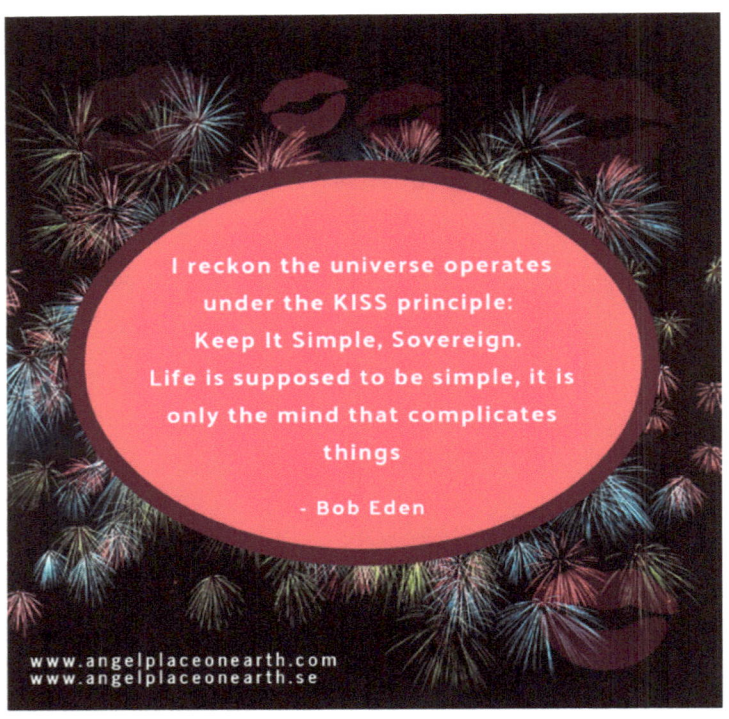

I reckon the universe operates under the KISS principle:
Keep It Simple, Sovereign.
Life is supposed to be simple, it is only the mind that complicates things

- Bob Eden

www.angelplaceonearth.com
www.angelplaceonearth.se

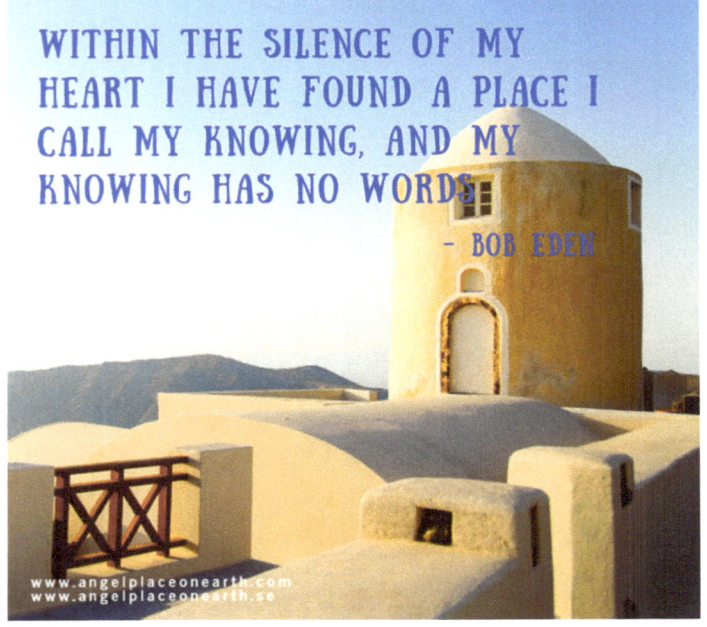

WITHIN THE SILENCE OF MY HEART I HAVE FOUND A PLACE I CALL MY KNOWING, AND MY KNOWING HAS NO WORDS

- BOB EDEN

www.angelplaceonearth.com
www.angelplaceonearth.se

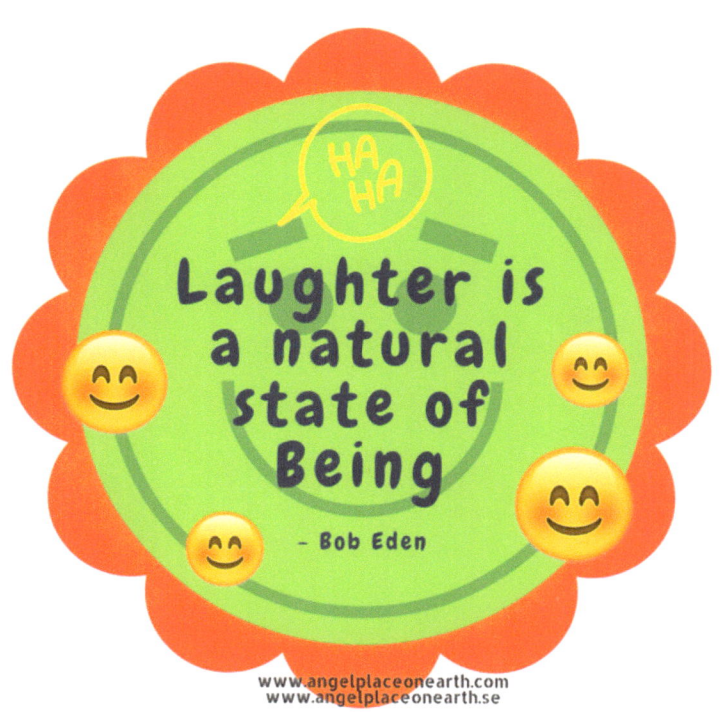

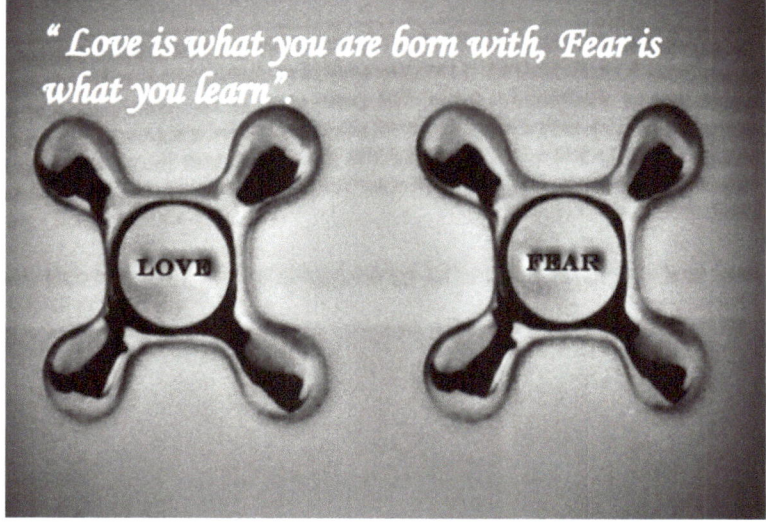

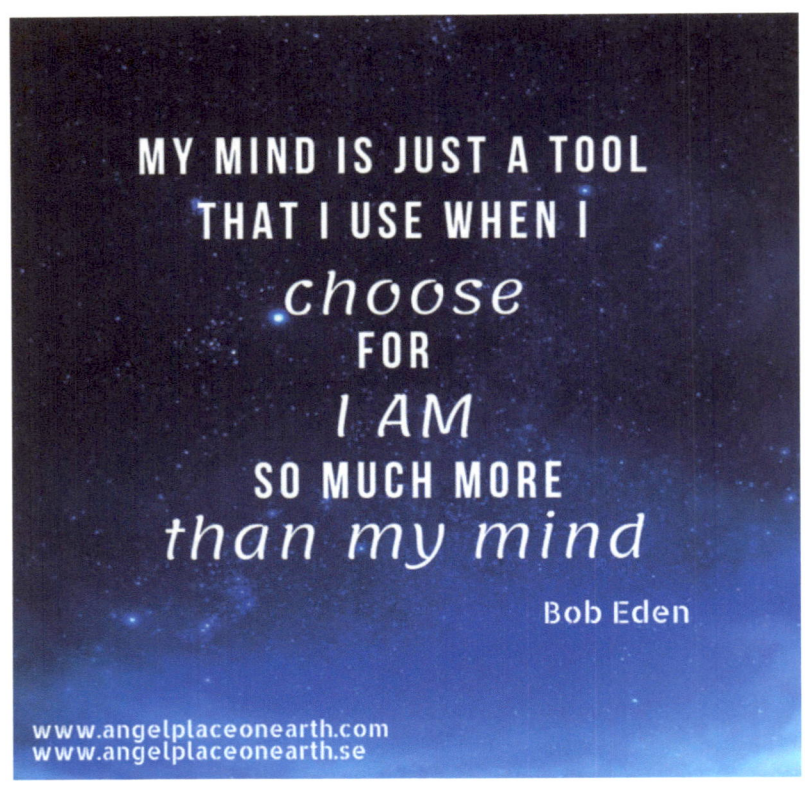

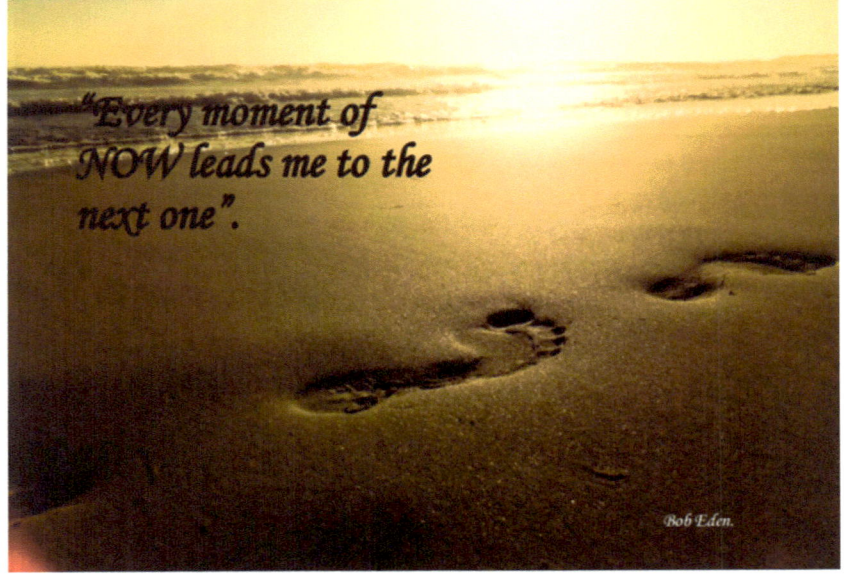

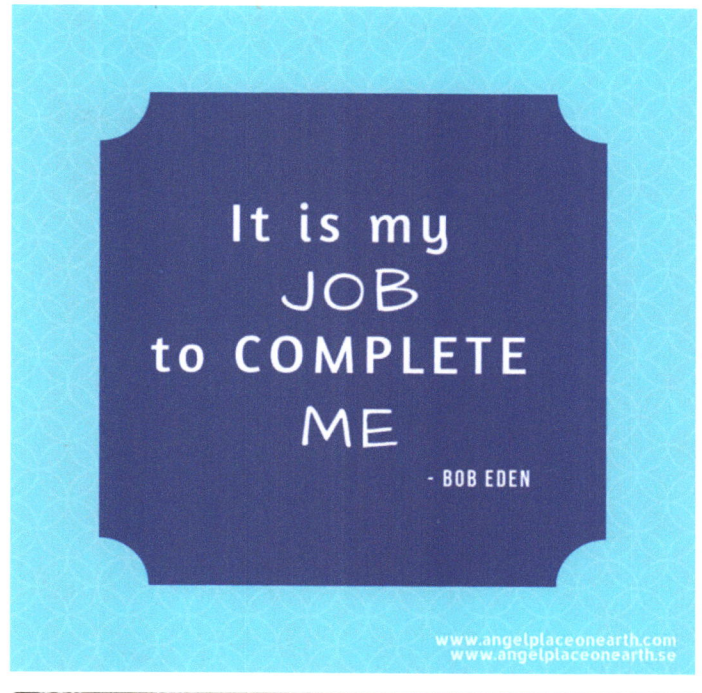

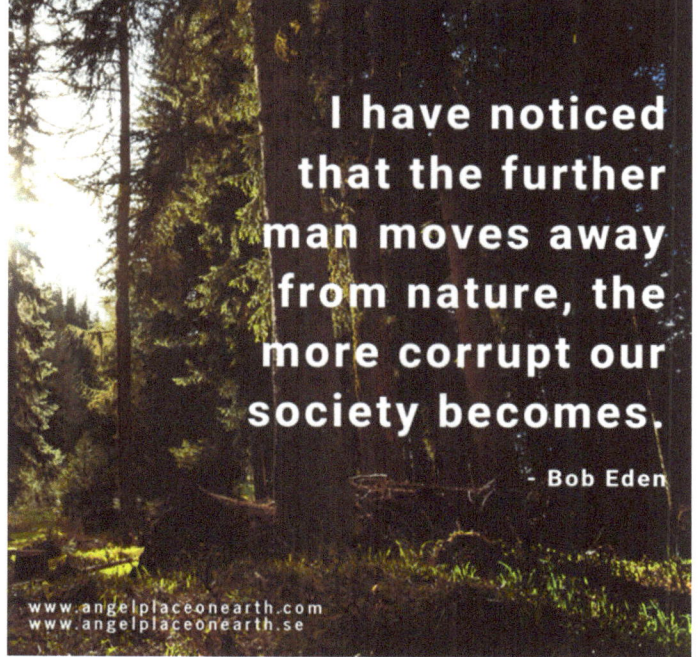

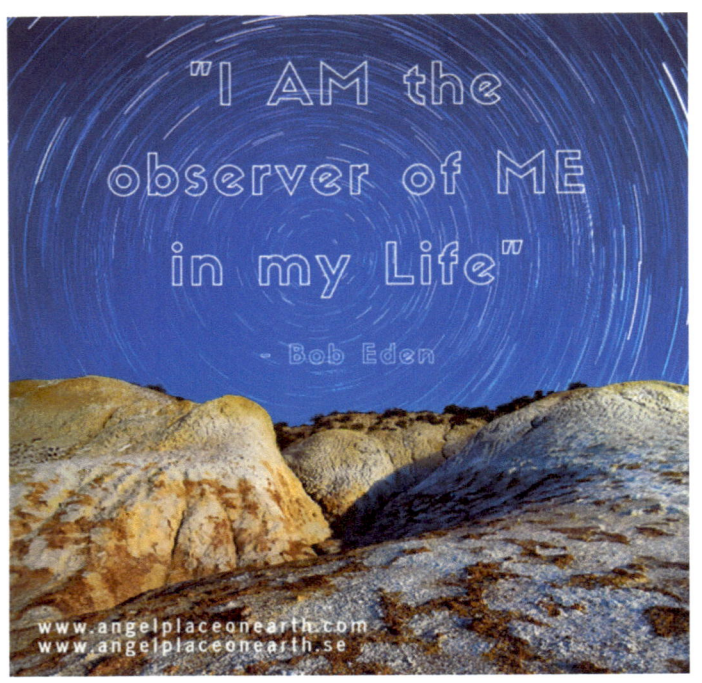

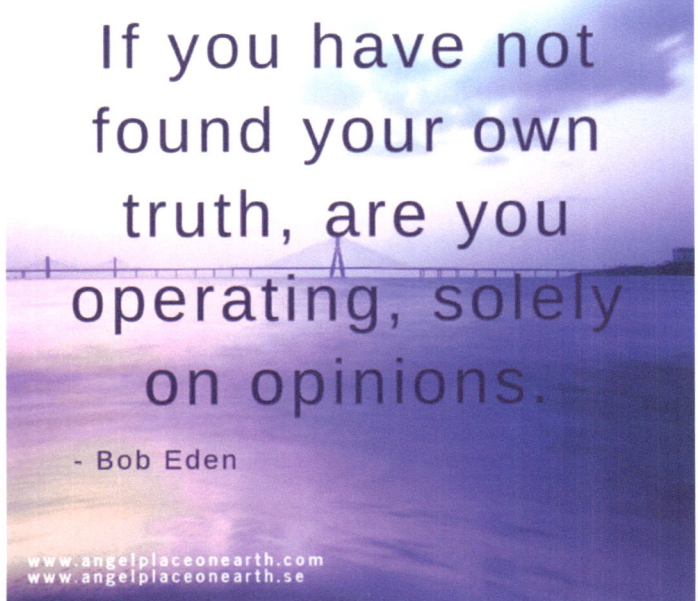

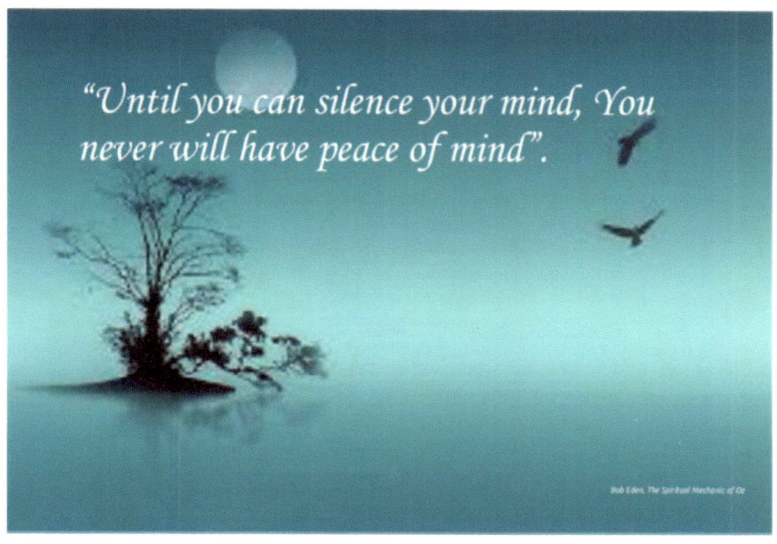

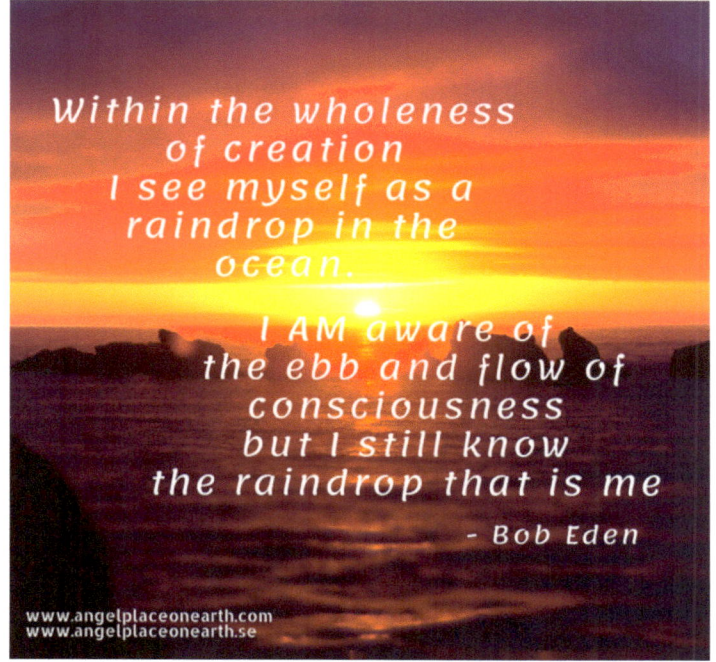

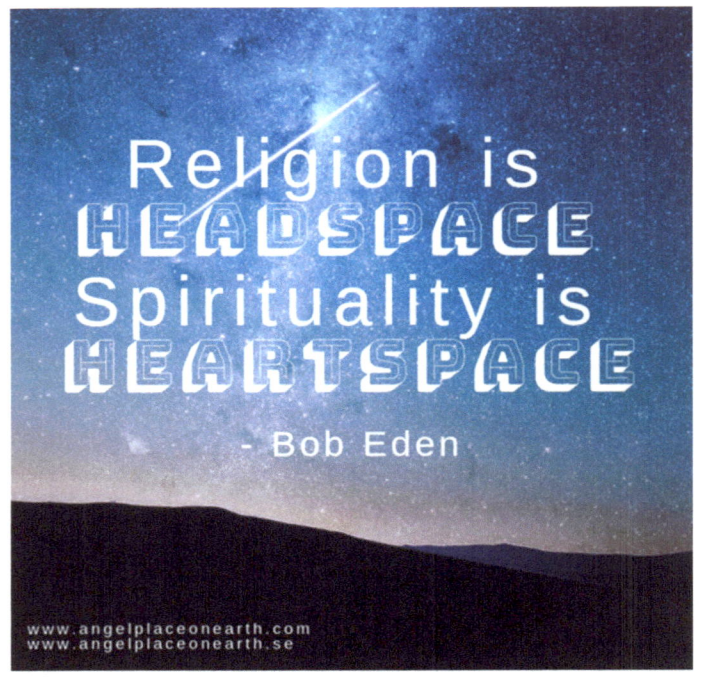

RESPECT YOURSELF
ENOUGH TO WALK
AWAY FROM
ANYTHING THAT
NO LONGER
SERVES YOU,
GROWS YOU OR
MAKES YOU HAPPY.

WWW.**LIVELIFEHAPPY**.COM

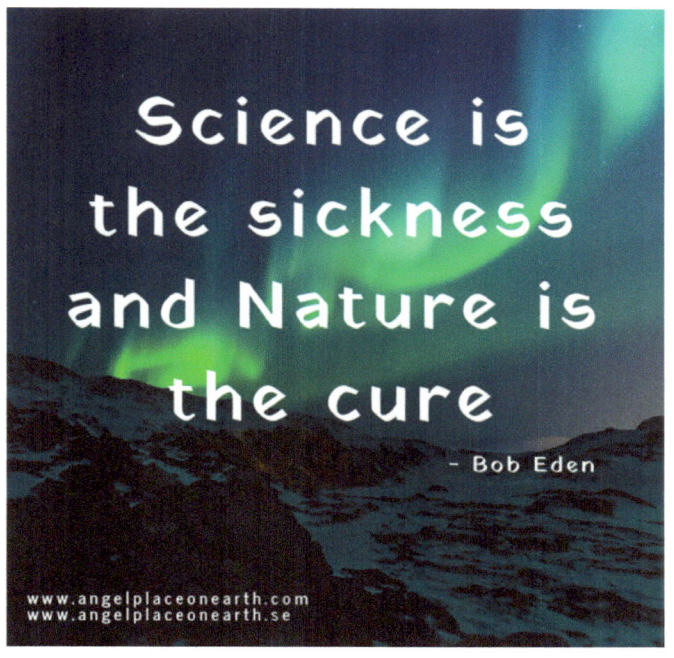

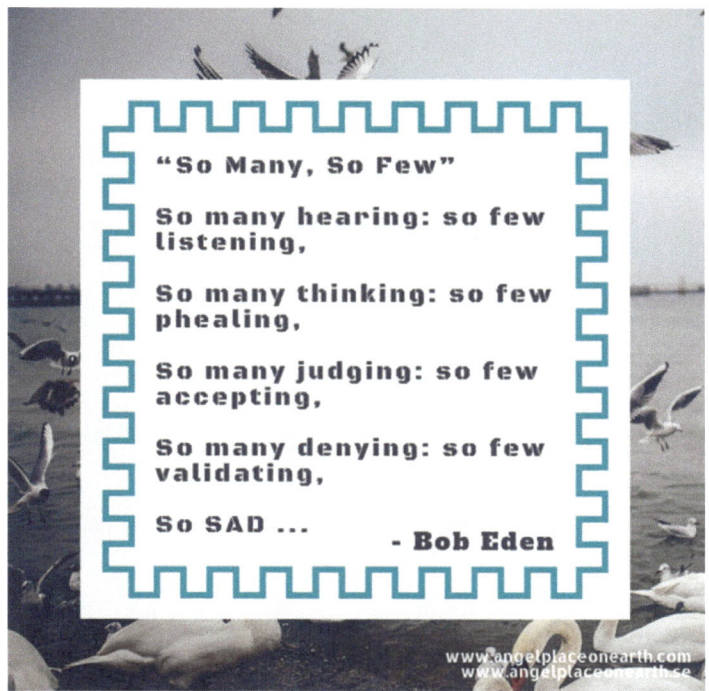

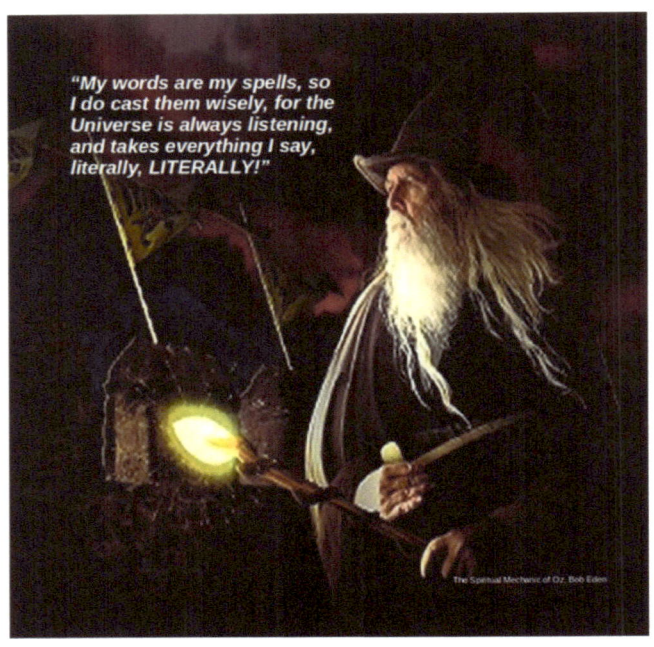

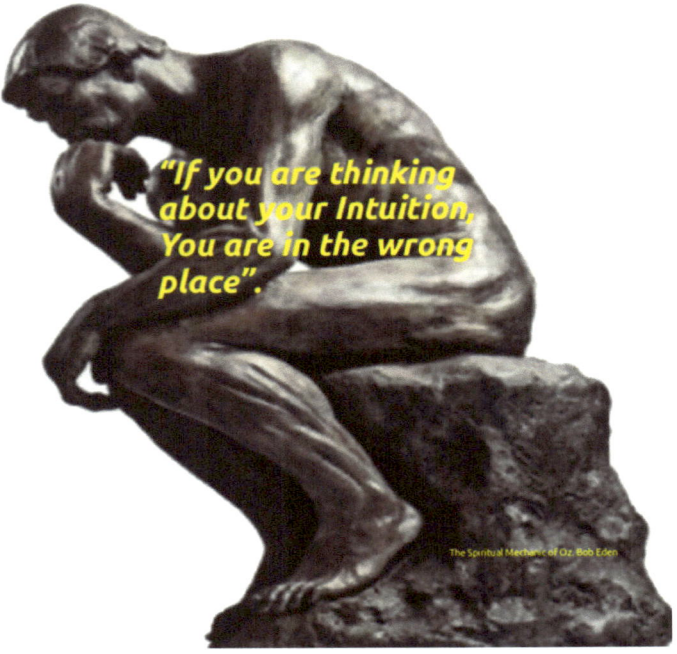

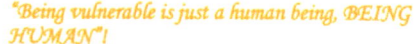

"Being vulnerable is just a human being, BEING HUMAN"!

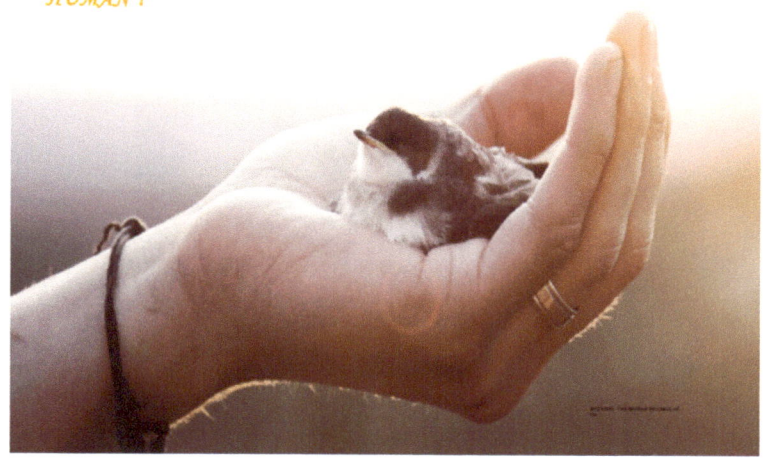

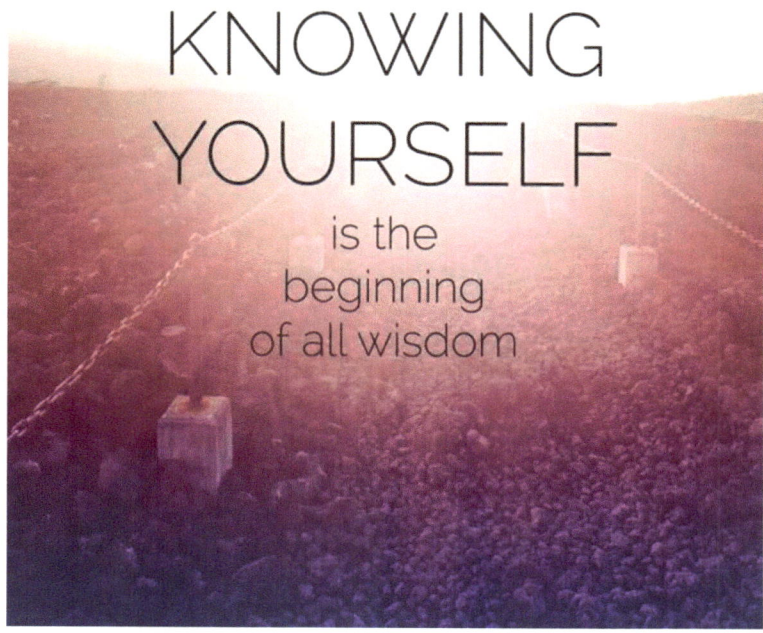

KNOWING YOURSELF is the beginning of all wisdom

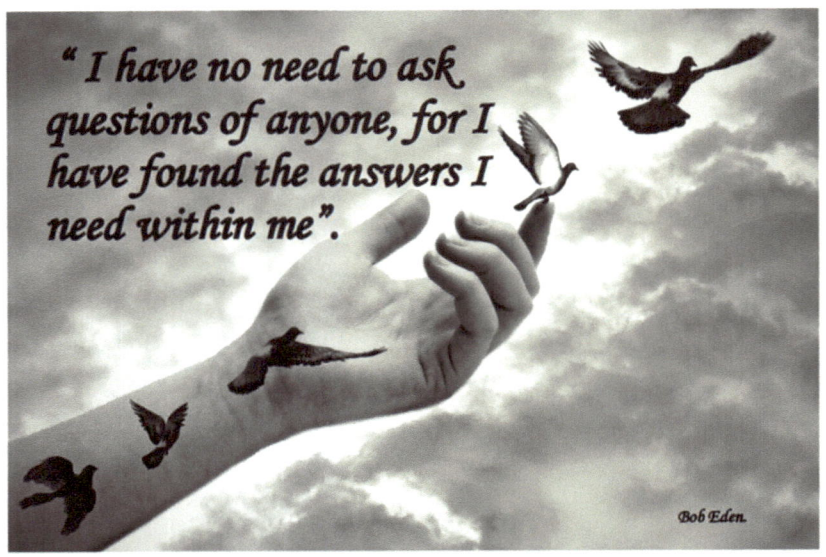

" I have no need to ask questions of anyone, for I have found the answers I need within me".

Bob Eden.

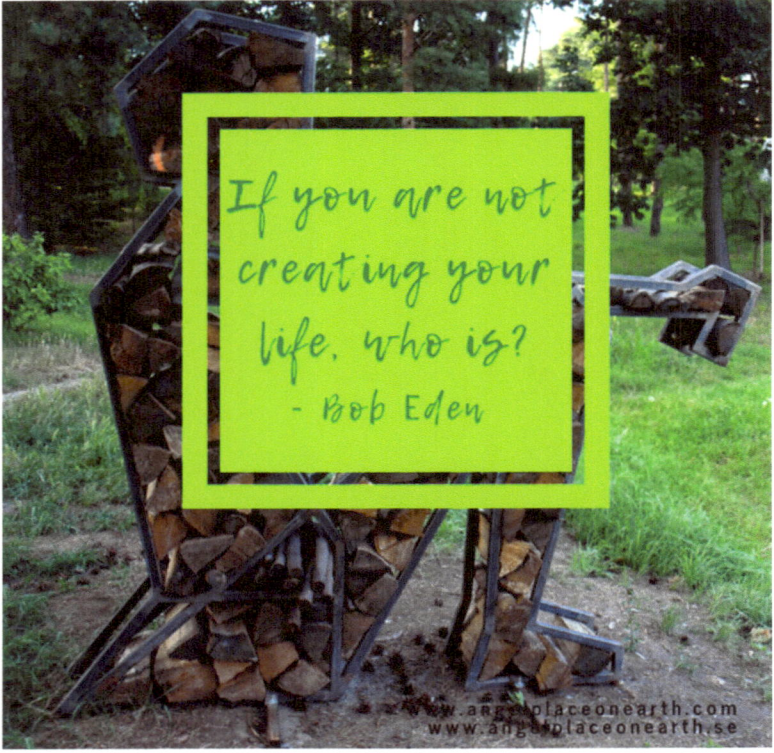

If you are not creating your life, who is?
- Bob Eden

www.angelplaceonearth.com
www.angelplaceonearth.se

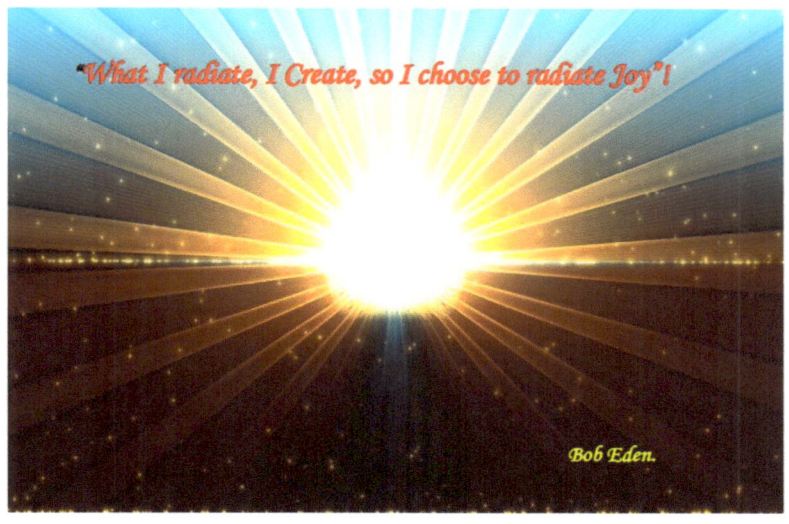

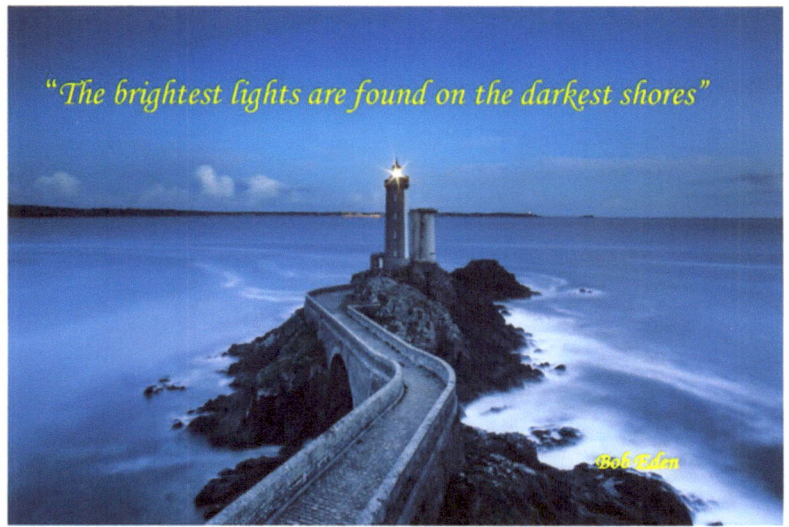

My favourite links

http://www.blogtalkradio.com/loveyouraddiction/2019/06/03/victim-or-victorwhat-do-you- choose

https://www.bitchute.com/video/clbsRyjpgP3k/no such thing as mental illness https://ochelli.com/the-gift-of-depression/ Bob Eden The Gift of depression. https://youtu.be/hdQeEnQ7h_A Cure for 97%, MMS.

https://youtu.be/mQc_-myy4ts running from the cure, Rick Simpson. https://youtu.be/qnxPWPAZ7Ds wakey wakey ep5. https://www.youtube.com/watch?v=t5eYncE4khQ the Mayan calendar comes north.

http://www.blogtalkradio.com/sierra-neblina/2016/11/08/becoming-a-cosmic-citizen--bob- eden--living-his-dream Bob Eden Living his dream.

http://www.blogtalkradio.com/naasca/20https://youtu.be/eOScYBwMyAA19/04/25/stop-child- abuse-now-scan--2123

https://youtu.be/Amvrvme4rBs MMS.

https://youtu.be/r0c9NTg17mQ can depression can be cured without medication. https://youtu.be/6iDMuB6NjNA the power listening.

https://youtu.be/W-r6sg1RQ0Y bark endeavour. https://www.bitchute.com/video/xdQt41It9nNW/ The Greatest story never told. https://

youtu.be/B44abxGmBYA Wayne Glew Constitution and Rights. https://youtu.be/U7HJI5Jwzt0 Wayne Glew

https://youtu.be/-4Lnze7O22g Pirates of the suburbs. https://youtu.be/hy5xOT3X38I my gift of depression. https://anchor.fm/bob-eden https://youtu.be/PAaWZTFRP9Q ken robinson and sadhguru

https://youtu.be/VMqcLUqYqrs the greatest 3 minutes in tv history.

https://www.transformationtalkradio.com/e/28340 gift of depression.

https://www.blogtalkradio.com/ysticalawakeningsradio/2020/02/05/sjr-bob-eden-the-gift-of-depression?fbclid=IwAR0_cPvJepa-cnjMql vbJQcrHm1Lr0v- c_oYScJ3l7krKxbOiEOroDiU2Bg

https://youtu.be/DonHR12gx7Y Kornelia Stephanie show G O D. https://youtu.be/SJUhlRoBL8M always look on the bright side of life. https://youtu.be/UBAAgdRHWlM John Bradshaw, Healing the shame that binds you. https://tombarnett.tv/2020/10/28/the-gift-of-depression-with-bob-eden-2/ https://youtu.be/WnWi8ljqUFo wounds and lessons of childhood Kris Kalea. https://www.bitchute.com/video/xlLRMnjNBQEO/ why you can't catch a virus. https://youtu.be/m-g8UbOH1kQ linsy helleger.

https://www.bitchute.com/video/WQ4yVUXy5xgN/ Catherine Edwards. https://www.youtube.com/watch?v=8b5srY9Y34U The Campfire Project. https://youtu.be/M8mfYyfjZmY The END of depression. https://youtu.be/aFWAXFmL8DY the end of depression with Catherine Edwards. https://earthheroestv.com/programs/bob-eden-heartspace-or-headspace?offset=3519 https://youtu.be/hmQ9PHIeU3A My Garden of Eden.

https://www.bitchute.com/video/kgyyG1AJMyl0/Knowing and Knowledge with Catherine Edwards.

Acknowledgements

Where do I start?

Well my #1 mentor was Barnaby, my little Tenterfield terrier. He and I were inseparable for 14 years,until his passing in June 2021. He taught me how to live in the NOW,and was always there to give counsel and support. RIP Barnaby!

Next would be John Bradshaw, and his work on the inner child and healing the shame that binds you, his work truly saved my life, so thankyou John RIP.

Ian Xel Lungold, for his work on The Mayan Calendar,

I felt as if I had been hit by a truck after watching his presentations on the Maya culture, they certainly put me in my place in the grand scheme of things, and sowed the seeds for many of the insights that I would discover later in my own journey. RIP Ian.

Val Hastings, A true earth angel and powerhouse. I had the pleasure of singing with her for many years. The joy she brought to my life and many others was and still is immeasurable . RIP Val.

Valeria Neu, who was my partner, soul mate and best friend during the darkest times of my depression, and who managed to capture my very essence in the pencil sketch that is the front cover for this book.

David Richards, a recent new friend, for his unfailing support to me in writing this book, I never knew how hard it was going to be, but David kept urging me along, so thankyou David.

I have had an amazing life, even with all that depression, and every step I have taken how ever good or bad, and every one I have met along the way has helped me to reach my own contentment.

"Apologies"

I'm no saint,

during my drugged era I found that every anti-depressant that I took turned me into some one I did not like and I behaved badly at times, so for those folks that I have hurt in the past, I would like to offer my heart felt apology, I hope that you are able to forgive me.

Thankfully those times are now long gone!

"The Future"

If my story has value for you and would like more information, just search the internet for:"Bob Eden The Gift of Depression".

If you would like to connect with me: Bob Eden on facebook or"authorbob@gmx.com", I would appreciate any comments, feed back or polite suggestions, hahaha!

I AM on a mission to eradicate suicide, and from what I know and what I FEEL, this is entirely doable! Wish me luck! You can help me achieve my mission by subscribing to my mailing list: https://bit.ly/bobaweber and my Youtube channel: https://bit.ly/3vOKprZ. Thankyou.

Until we meet again remember:" If you are not creating your life, WHO is?"

Much love from Bob and Charlie .

Bold Barnaby, my guide and mentor for 14 years who sadly is no longer here next to me.

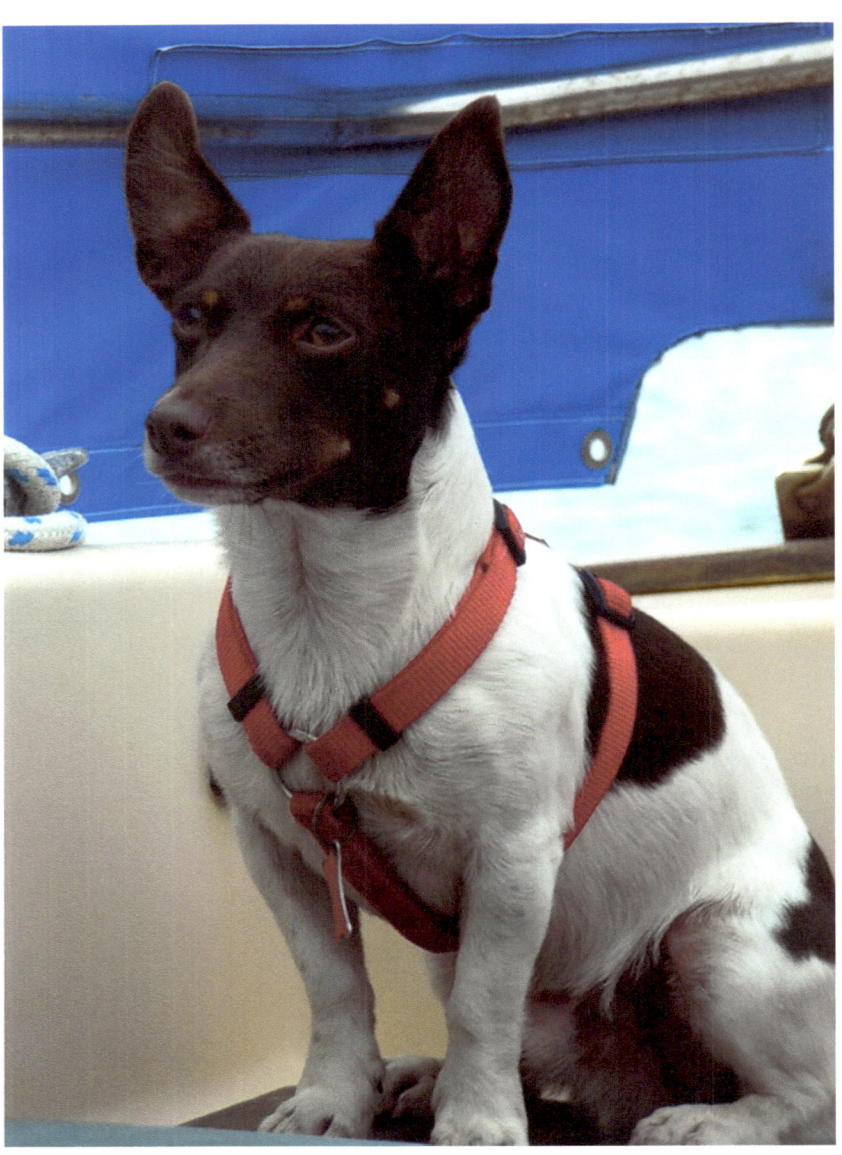

www.ingramcontent.com/pod-product-compliance
Lightning Source LLC
Chambersburg PA
CBHW040857120626
46551CB00001B/55